Anatomical Visual Guide to

Sports Injuries

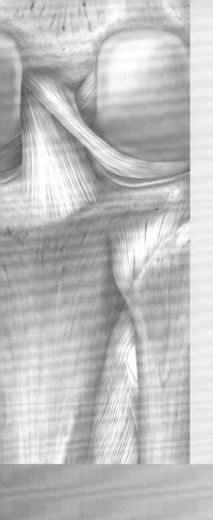

Contents

Each chapter in this guide is devoted to a specific region of the body, starting with Head and Neck and ending with Foot and Ankle. Because anatomy is the foundation for any sports medicine clinician, each section includes detailed images of anatomy—mainly of adults, however pediatric growth plate visuals can be found in certain sections. Chapters also include visual images of movement, injuries, and examples of the mechanism of select injuries. Bonus anatomical system charts are also included after the last section.

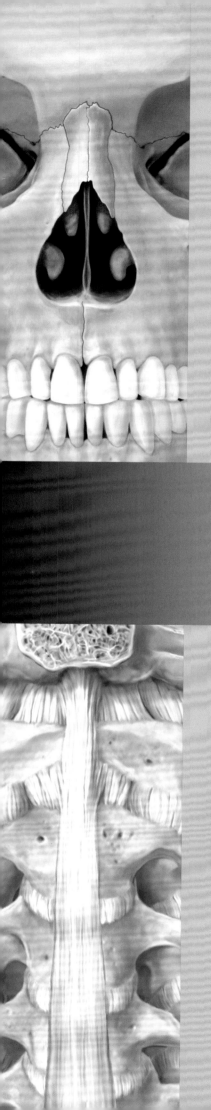

Head and Neck

Nerve Central

The head and neck house the body's complex nerve centers, and as a result, injuries to these areas can have the most catastrophic consequences. Collision sports such as hockey, rugby and football are at an increased risk for injury, but so are sports that place an athlete at height such as cheerleading, gymnastics and diving. Injury to the head and neck often occurs simultaneously, and requires careful monitoring and a solid recognition of common injury mechanisms.

chapter

1

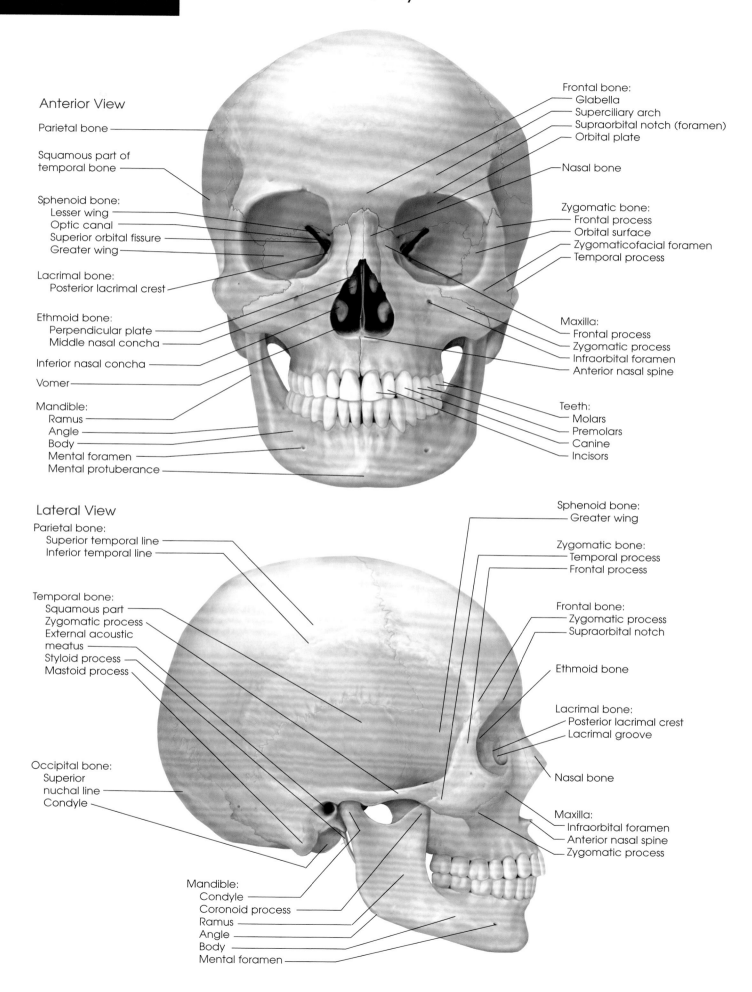

Anterior View

Parietal bone

Squamous part of
temporal bone

Sphenoid bone:
Lesser wing
Optic canal
Superior orbital fissure
Greater wing

Lacrimal bone:
Posterior lacrimal crest

Ethmoid bone:
Perpendicular plate
Middle nasal concha

Inferior nasal concha

Vomer

Mandible:
Ramus
Angle
Body
Mental foramen
Mental protuberance

Frontal bone:
Glabella
Superciliary arch
Supraorbital notch (foramen)
Orbital plate

Nasal bone

Zygomatic bone:
Frontal process
Orbital surface
Zygomaticofacial foramen
Temporal process

Maxilla:
Frontal process
Zygomatic process
Infraorbital foramen
Anterior nasal spine

Teeth:
Molars
Premolars
Canine
Incisors

Lateral View

Parietal bone:
Superior temporal line
Inferior temporal line

Temporal bone:
Squamous part
Zygomatic process
External acoustic
meatus
Styloid process
Mastoid process

Occipital bone:
Superior
nuchal line
Condyle

Mandible:
Condyle
Coronoid process
Ramus
Angle
Body
Mental foramen

Sphenoid bone:
Greater wing

Zygomatic bone:
Temporal process
Frontal process

Frontal bone:
Zygomatic process
Supraorbital notch

Ethmoid bone

Lacrimal bone:
Posterior lacrimal crest
Lacrimal groove

Nasal bone

Maxilla:
Infraorbital foramen
Anterior nasal spine
Zygomatic process

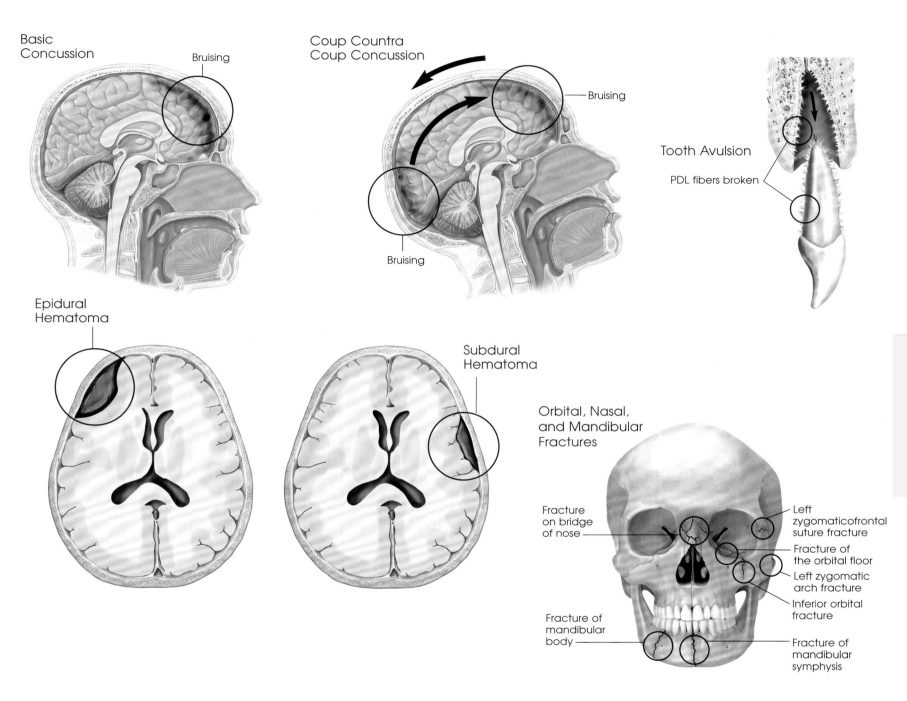

Basic
Concussion

Bruising

Coup Countra
Coup Concussion

Bruising

Bruising

Tooth Avulsion

PDL fibers broken

Epidural
Hematoma

Subdural
Hematoma

Orbital, Nasal,
and Mandibular
Fractures

Fracture
on bridge
of nose

Left
zygomaticofrontal
suture fracture

Fracture of
the orbital floor

Left zygomatic
arch fracture

Inferior orbital
fracture

Fracture of
mandibular
body

Fracture of
mandibular
symphysis

Mechanism of Injury

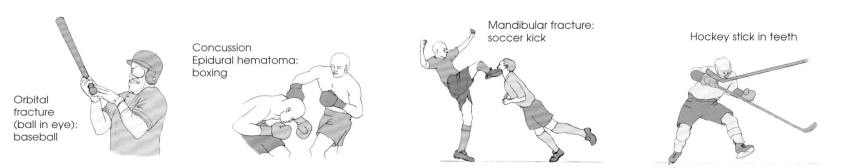

Mandibular fracture:
soccer kick

Hockey stick in teeth

Concussion
Epidural hematoma:
boxing

Orbital
fracture
(ball in eye):
baseball

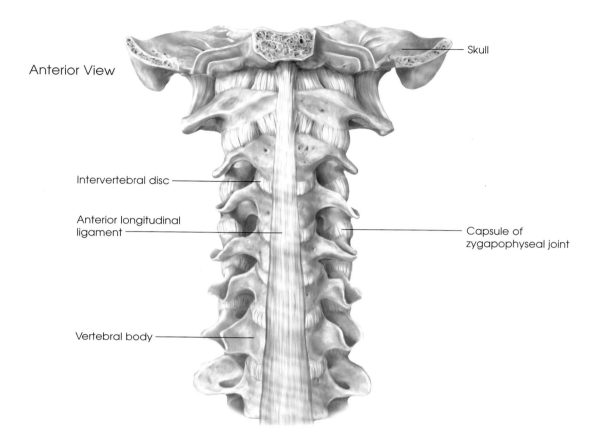

Anterior View

Intervertebral disc

Anterior longitudinal ligament

Vertebral body

Skull

Capsule of zygapophyseal joint

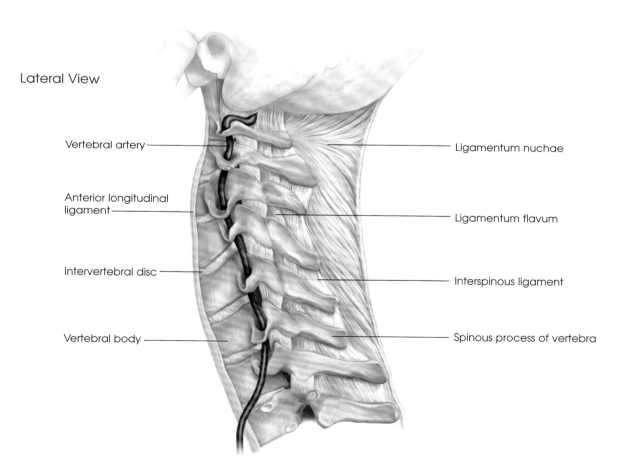

Lateral View

Vertebral artery

Anterior longitudinal ligament

Intervertebral disc

Vertebral body

Ligamentum nuchae

Ligamentum flavum

Interspinous ligament

Spinous process of vertebra

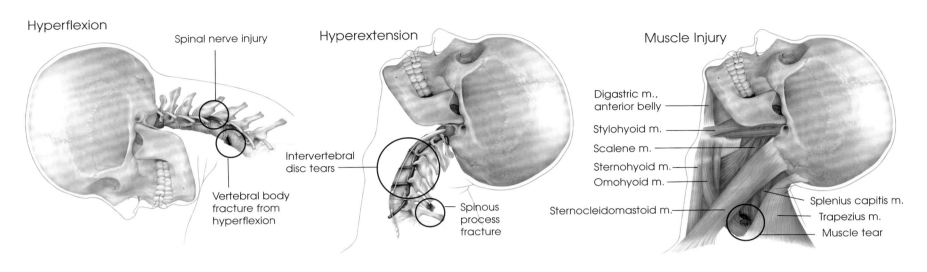

Hyperflexion

Spinal nerve injury

Vertebral body fracture from hyperflexion

Hyperextension

Intervertebral disc tears

Spinous process fracture

Muscle Injury

Digastric m., anterior belly

Stylohyoid m.

Scalene m.

Sternohyoid m.

Omohyoid m.

Sternocleidomastoid m.

Splenius capitis m.

Trapezius m.

Muscle tear

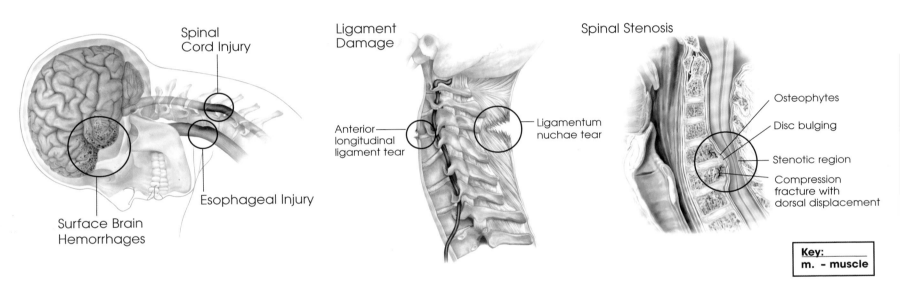

Spinal Cord Injury

Surface Brain Hemorrhages

Esophageal Injury

Ligament Damage

Anterior longitudinal ligament tear

Ligamentum nuchae tear

Spinal Stenosis

Osteophytes

Disc bulging

Stenotic region

Compression fracture with dorsal displacement

Key:
m. – muscle

Movements

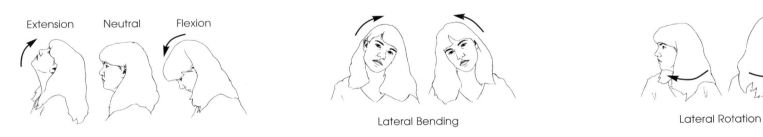

Extension   Neutral   Flexion

Lateral Bending

Lateral Rotation

Mechanism of Injury

Burner and stinger: football

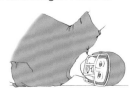

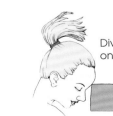
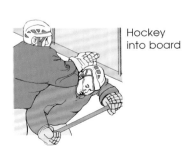
Hockey into board

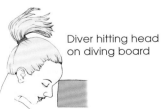
Diver hitting head on diving board

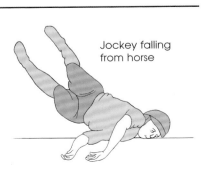
Jockey falling from horse

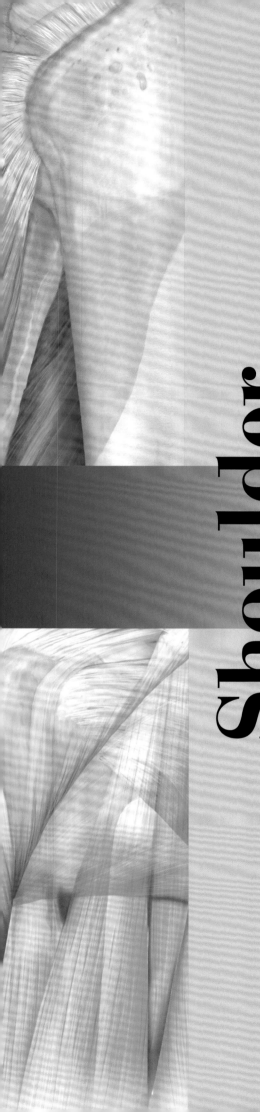

Shoulder

A Key Player

The shoulder joint is one of the most important joints in sports as its broad range of motion allows the athlete to perform many feats. Unfortunately, the benefit of mobility combined with the repetitive overhead and cocking motions required in sports like tennis and baseball, place this joint at risk of dislocation and tears. Understanding the complex relationship between the scapula, rotator cuff and glenohumeral joint is necessary to provide optimal care.

chapter 2

Anterior View

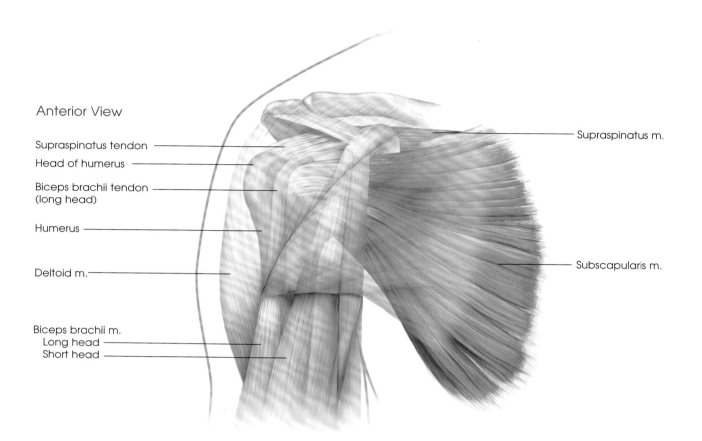

Supraspinatus tendon

Head of humerus

Biceps brachii tendon
(long head)

Humerus

Deltoid m.

Biceps brachii m.
Long head
Short head

Supraspinatus m.

Subscapularis m.

Superolateral View

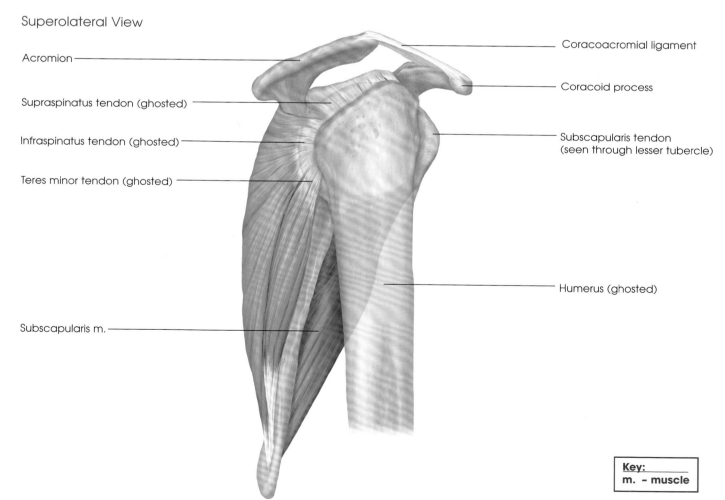

Acromion

Supraspinatus tendon (ghosted)

Infraspinatus tendon (ghosted)

Teres minor tendon (ghosted)

Subscapularis m.

Coracoacromial ligament

Coracoid process

Subscapularis tendon
(seen through lesser tubercle)

Humerus (ghosted)

Key:
m. – muscle

Impingement and Biceps Problems

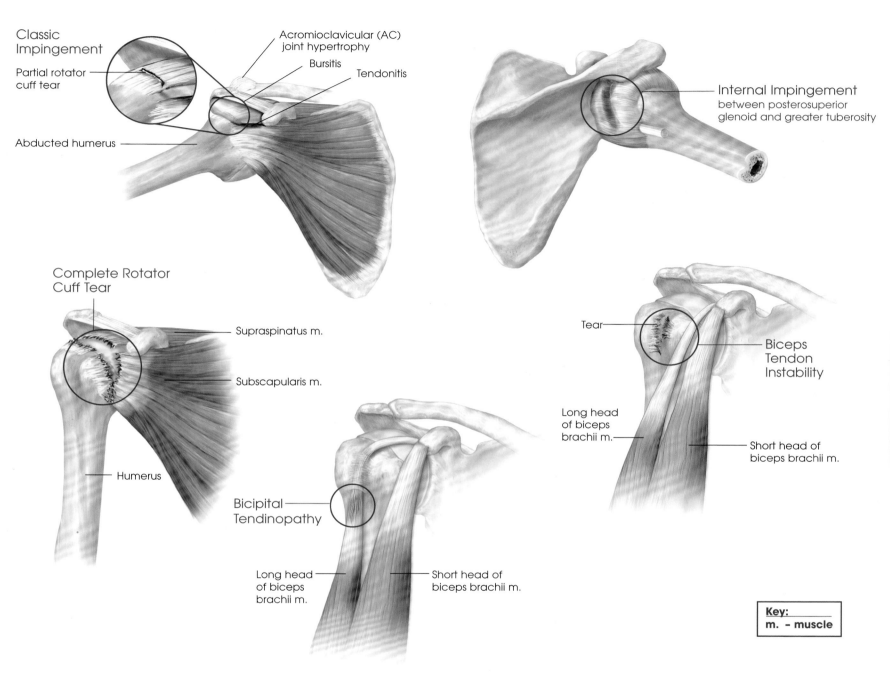

Classic Impingement

Partial rotator cuff tear

Abducted humerus

Acromioclavicular (AC) joint hypertrophy

Bursitis

Tendonitis

Internal Impingement
between posterosuperior glenoid and greater tuberosity

Complete Rotator Cuff Tear

Supraspinatus m.

Subscapularis m.

Humerus

Tear

Biceps Tendon Instability

Long head of biceps brachii m.

Short head of biceps brachii m.

Bicipital Tendinopathy

Long head of biceps brachii m.

Short head of biceps brachii m.

Key:
m. – muscle

Movements

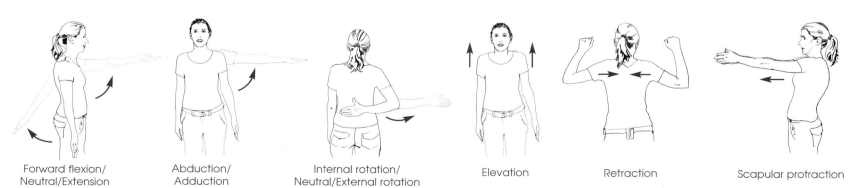

Forward flexion/ Neutral/Extension

Abduction/ Adduction

Internal rotation/ Neutral/External rotation

Elevation

Retraction

Scapular protraction

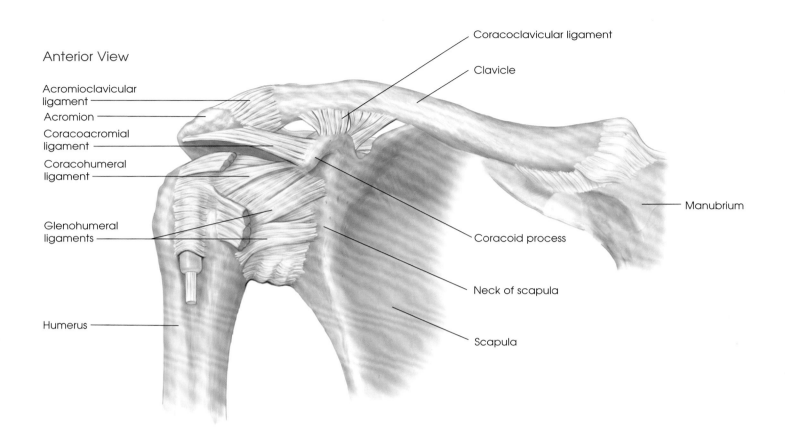

Anterior View

Coracoclavicular ligament

Clavicle

Acromioclavicular ligament

Acromion

Coracoacromial ligament

Coracohumeral ligament

Glenohumeral ligaments

Humerus

Manubrium

Coracoid process

Neck of scapula

Scapula

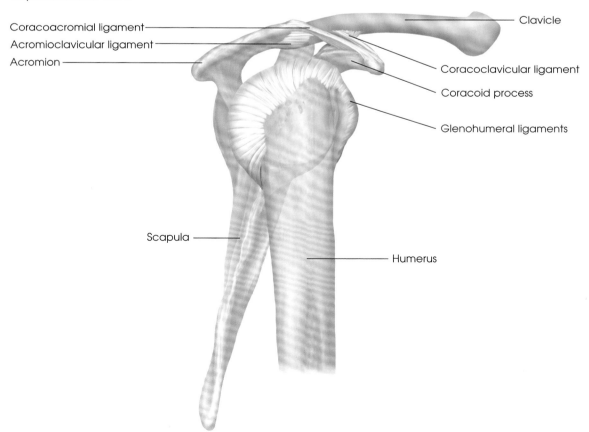

Superolateral View

Coracoacromial ligament

Acromioclavicular ligament

Acromion

Clavicle

Coracoclavicular ligament

Coracoid process

Glenohumeral ligaments

Scapula

Humerus

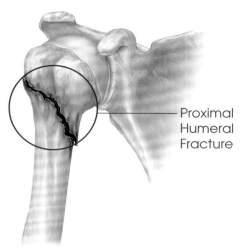

Proximal
Humeral
Fracture

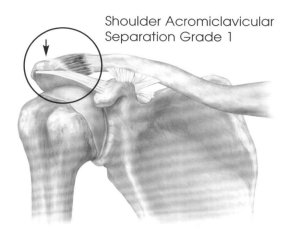

Shoulder Acromiclavicular
Separation Grade 1

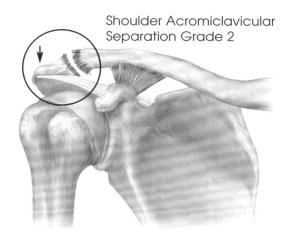

Shoulder Acromiclavicular
Separation Grade 2

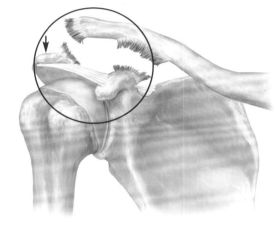

Shoulder Acromiclavicular
Separation Grade 3

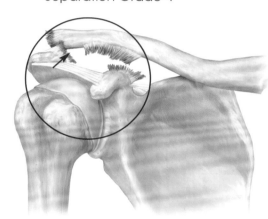

Shoulder Acromiclavicular
Separation Grade 4

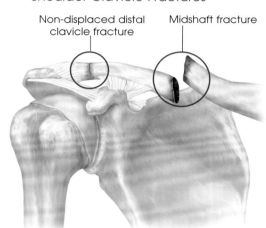

Shoulder Clavicle Fractures

Non-displaced distal
clavicle fracture

Midshaft fracture

Movements

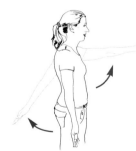

Forward flexion/
Neutral/Extension

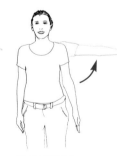

Abduction/
Adduction

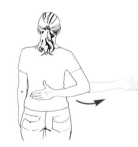

Internal rotation/
Neutral/External rotation

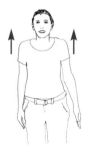

Elevation

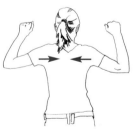

Retraction

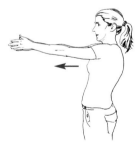

Scapular protraction

Mechanism of Injury

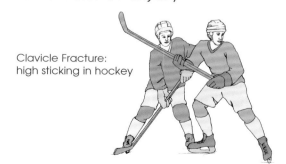

Clavicle Fracture:
high sticking in hockey

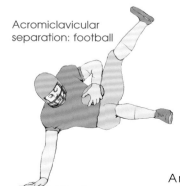

Acromiclavicular
separation: football

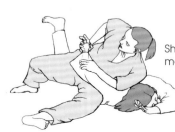

Shoulder dislocation:
martial arts

Normal Anatomy–
Growth Plates and Ossification Sites

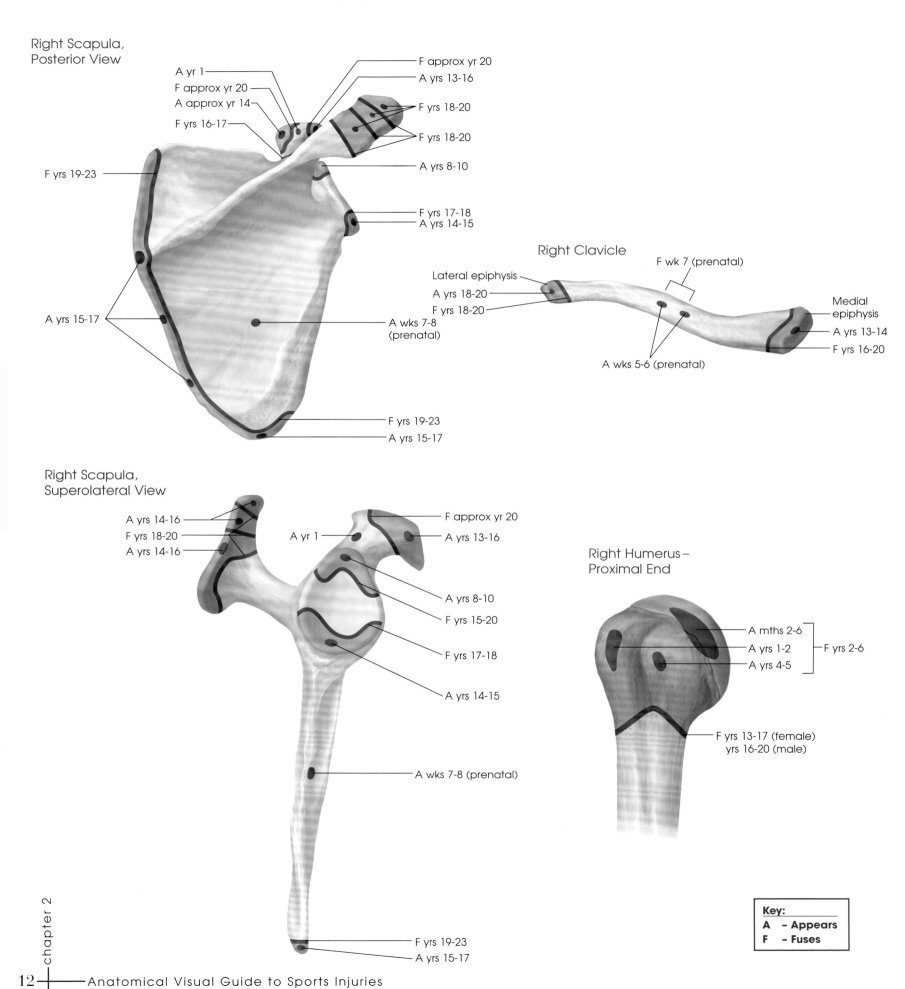

Right Scapula,
Posterior View

A yr 1
F approx yr 20
A approx yr 14
F yrs 16-17

F approx yr 20
A yrs 13-16
F yrs 18-20
F yrs 18-20

A yrs 8-10

F yrs 19-23

F yrs 17-18
A yrs 14-15

Right Clavicle

Lateral epiphysis
A yrs 18-20
F yrs 18-20

F wk 7 (prenatal)

Medial
epiphysis

A yrs 13-14
F yrs 16-20

A wks 5-6 (prenatal)

A yrs 15-17

A wks 7-8
(prenatal)

F yrs 19-23
A yrs 15-17

Right Scapula,
Superolateral View

A yrs 14-16
F yrs 18-20
A yrs 14-16

A yr 1

F approx yr 20
A yrs 13-16

A yrs 8-10
F yrs 15-20

F yrs 17-18

A yrs 14-15

A wks 7-8 (prenatal)

Right Humerus–
Proximal End

A mths 2-6
A yrs 1-2
A yrs 4-5

F yrs 2-6

F yrs 13-17 (female)
yrs 16-20 (male)

F yrs 19-23
A yrs 15-17

Key:
A – Appears
F – Fuses

Acromion

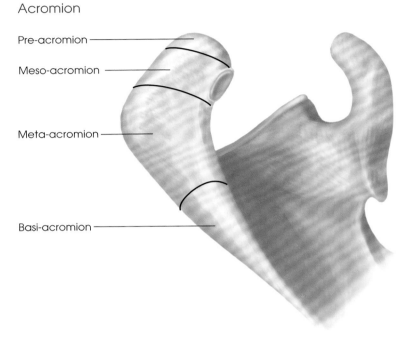

Pre-acromion

Meso-acromion

Meta-acromion

Basi-acromion

Little Leaguer's Shoulder
(Proximal Physis)

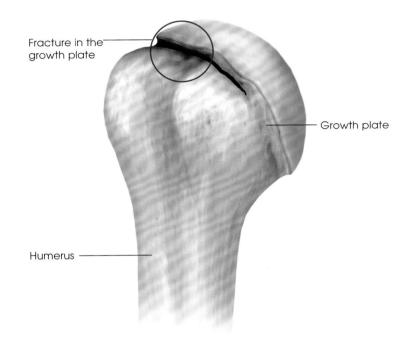

Fracture in the
growth plate

Growth plate

Humerus

Movements

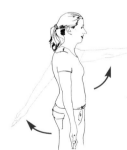

Forward flexion/
Neutral/extension

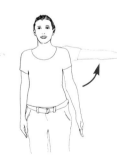

Abduction/
Neutral/adduction

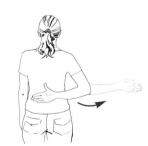

Internal rotation/
Neutral/External rotation

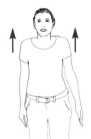

Elevation

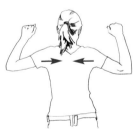

Retraction

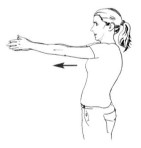

Scapular protraction

Mechanism of Injury

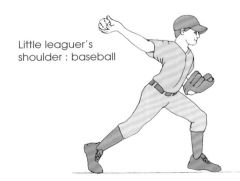

Little leaguer's
shoulder : baseball

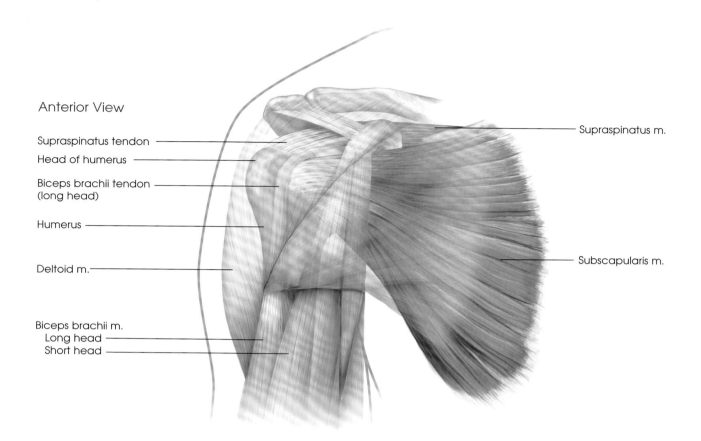

Anterior View

Supraspinatus tendon

Head of humerus

Biceps brachii tendon
(long head)

Humerus

Deltoid m.

Biceps brachii m.
Long head
Short head

Supraspinatus m.

Subscapularis m.

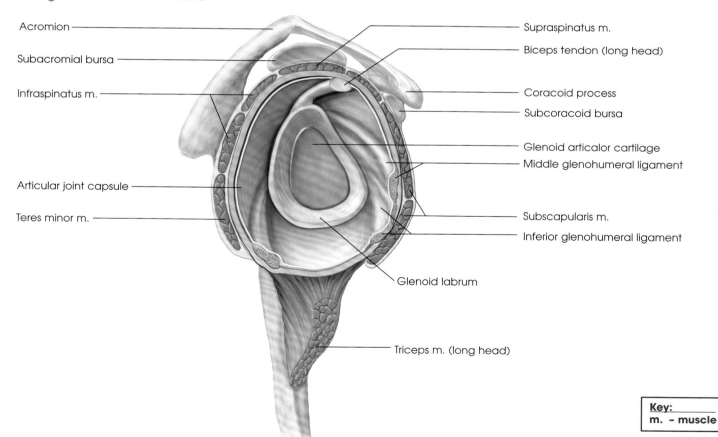

Lateral View
of Right Shoulder Joint Socket

Acromion

Subacromial bursa

Infraspinatus m.

Articular joint capsule

Teres minor m.

Supraspinatus m.

Biceps tendon (long head)

Coracoid process

Subcoracoid bursa

Glenoid articalor cartilage

Middle glenohumeral ligament

Subscapularis m.

Inferior glenohumeral ligament

Glenoid labrum

Triceps m. (long head)

Key:
m. – muscle

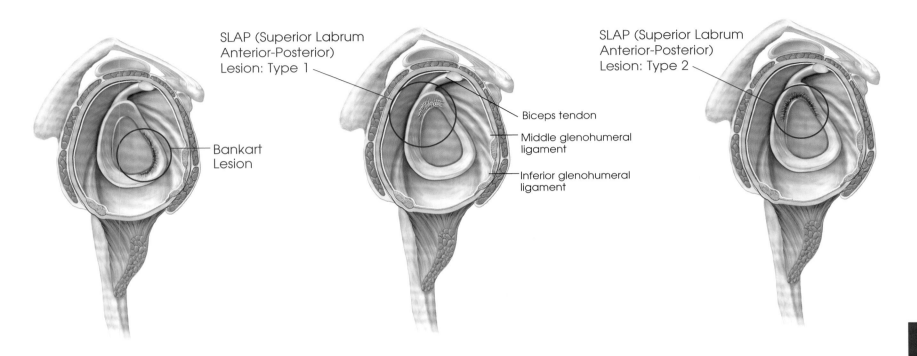

SLAP (Superior Labrum Anterior-Posterior) Lesion: Type 1

SLAP (Superior Labrum Anterior-Posterior) Lesion: Type 2

Biceps tendon

Middle glenohumeral ligament

Inferior glenohumeral ligament

Bankart Lesion

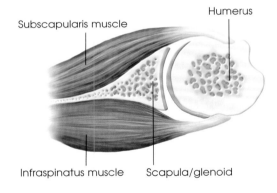

Normal Shoulder Anatomy

Subscapularis muscle

Humerus

Infraspinatus muscle

Scapula/glenoid

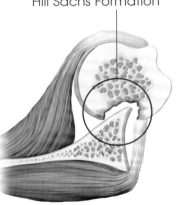

Anterior Dislocation with Hill Sachs Formation

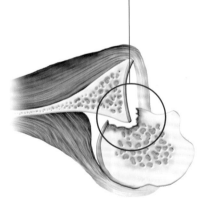

Posterior Dislocation with Reverse Hill Sachs Formation

Mechanism of Injury ──

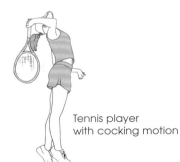

Tennis player with cocking motion

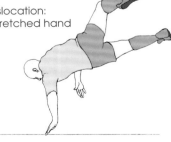

Shoulder dislocation: fall on outstretched hand in soccer

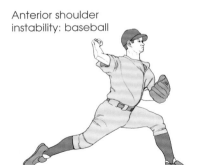

Anterior shoulder instability: baseball

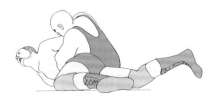

Anterior shoulder dislocation: wrestling

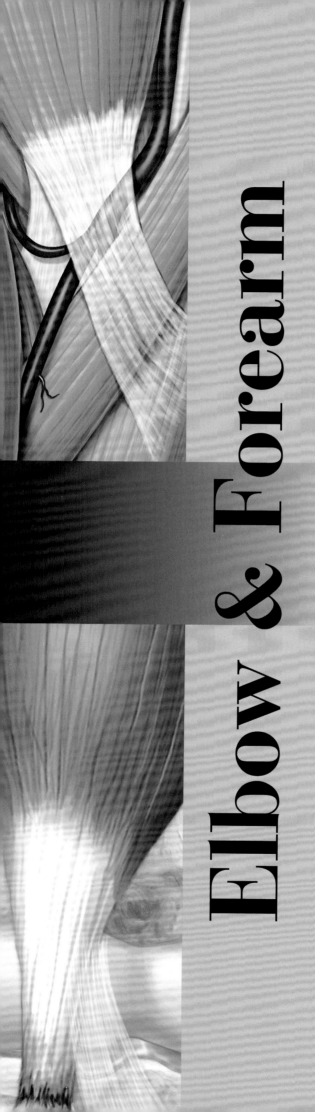

Elbow & Forearm

The Important Hinge

The elbow joint provides an important connection between the central core and the hand, which serves as the active delivery mechanism in most athletic activities. The elbow transfers loads and is at particular risk of injury caused by overuse in sports such as baseball, golf, and tennis. Knowledge of anatomy, development and common mechanisms of injury are vital to help prevent and treat elbow injury.

chapter 3

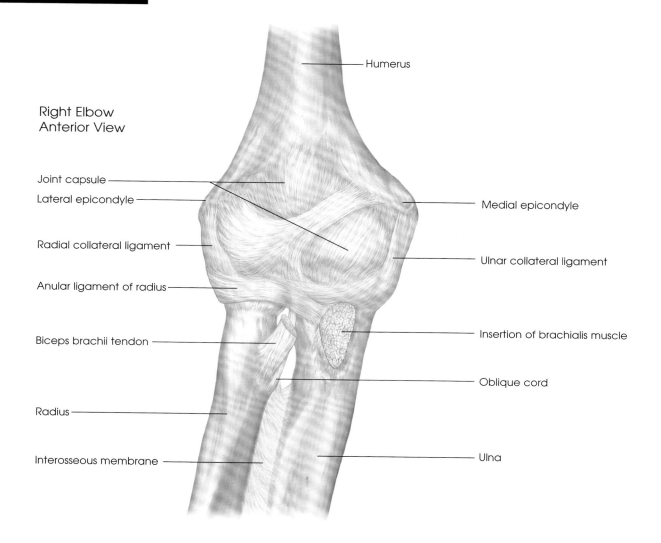

Right Elbow
Anterior View

Humerus

Joint capsule

Lateral epicondyle

Medial epicondyle

Radial collateral ligament

Ulnar collateral ligament

Anular ligament of radius

Biceps brachii tendon

Insertion of brachialis muscle

Oblique cord

Radius

Interosseous membrane

Ulna

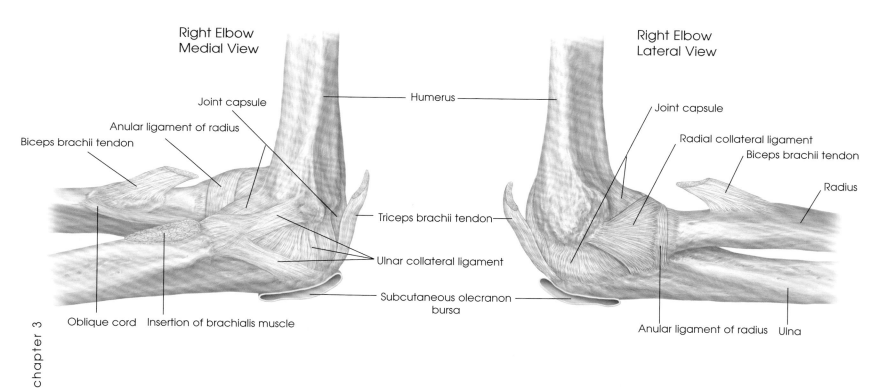

Right Elbow
Medial View

Right Elbow
Lateral View

Joint capsule

Anular ligament of radius

Biceps brachii tendon

Humerus

Joint capsule

Radial collateral ligament

Biceps brachii tendon

Radius

Triceps brachii tendon

Ulnar collateral ligament

Subcutaneous olecranon
bursa

Oblique cord   Insertion of brachialis muscle

Anular ligament of radius   Ulna

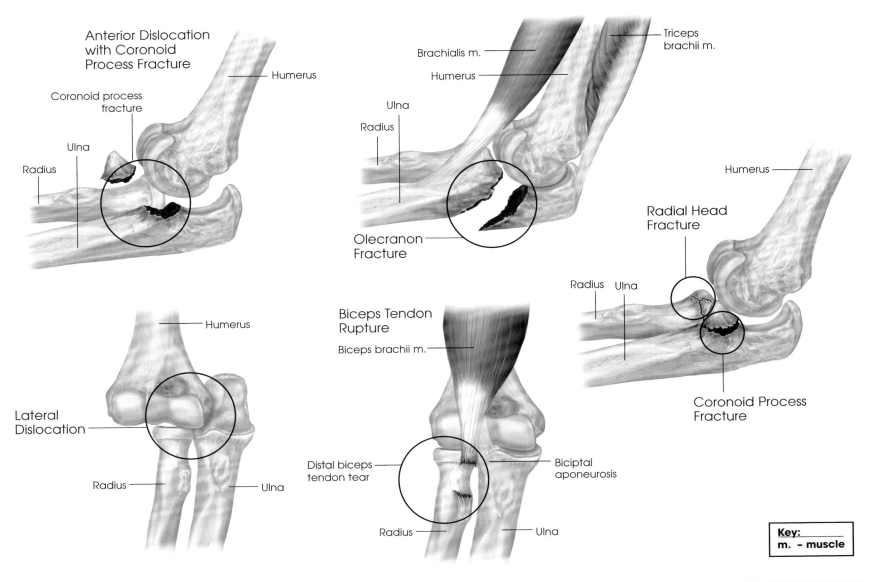

Anterior Dislocation with Coronoid Process Fracture

Coronoid process fracture

Ulna

Radius

Humerus

Brachialis m.

Humerus

Triceps brachii m.

Ulna

Radius

Olecranon Fracture

Humerus

Radial Head Fracture

Radius   Ulna

Coronoid Process Fracture

Humerus

Lateral Dislocation

Radius

Ulna

Biceps Tendon Rupture

Biceps brachii m.

Distal biceps tendon tear

Biciptal aponeurosis

Radius

Ulna

Key:
m. – muscle

Movements

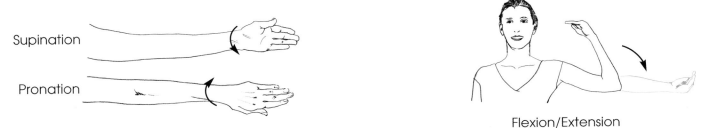

Supination

Pronation

Flexion/Extension

Mechanism of Injury

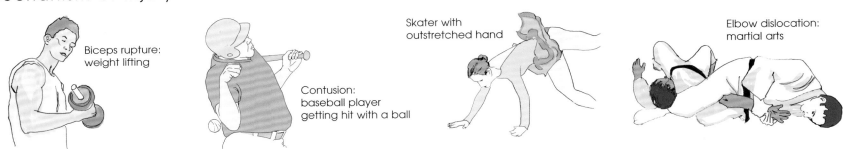

Biceps rupture: weight lifting

Contusion: baseball player getting hit with a ball

Skater with outstretched hand

Elbow dislocation: martial arts

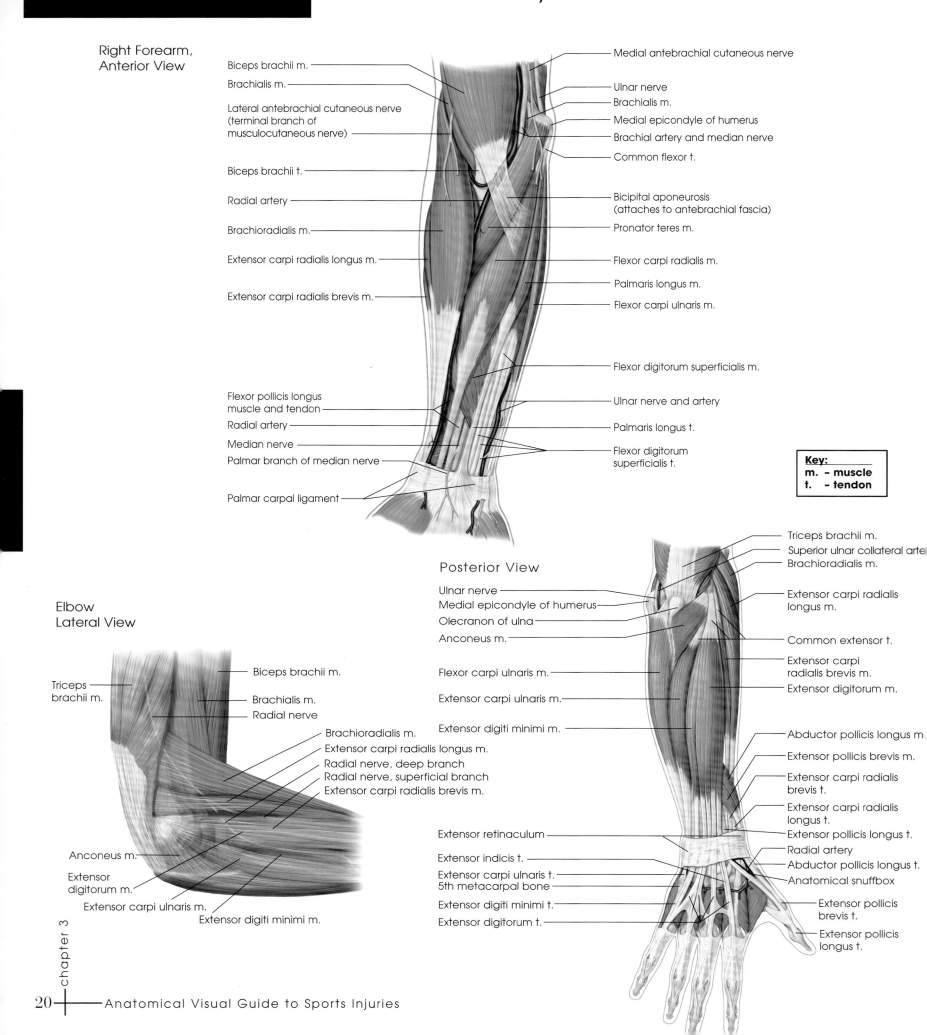

Right Forearm, Anterior View

Biceps brachii m.
Brachialis m.
Lateral antebrachial cutaneous nerve (terminal branch of musculocutaneous nerve)
Biceps brachii t.
Radial artery
Brachioradialis m.
Extensor carpi radialis longus m.
Extensor carpi radialis brevis m.
Flexor pollicis longus muscle and tendon
Radial artery
Median nerve
Palmar branch of median nerve
Palmar carpal ligament

Medial antebrachial cutaneous nerve
Ulnar nerve
Brachialis m.
Medial epicondyle of humerus
Brachial artery and median nerve
Common flexor t.
Bicipital aponeurosis (attaches to antebrachial fascia)
Pronator teres m.
Flexor carpi radialis m.
Palmaris longus m.
Flexor carpi ulnaris m.
Flexor digitorum superficialis m.
Ulnar nerve and artery
Palmaris longus t.
Flexor digitorum superficialis t.

Key:
m. – muscle
t. – tendon

Elbow Lateral View

Triceps brachii m.
Anconeus m.
Extensor digitorum m.
Extensor carpi ulnaris m.

Biceps brachii m.
Brachialis m.
Radial nerve
Brachioradialis m.
Extensor carpi radialis longus m.
Radial nerve, deep branch
Radial nerve, superficial branch
Extensor carpi radialis brevis m.
Extensor digiti minimi m.

Posterior View

Ulnar nerve
Medial epicondyle of humerus
Olecranon of ulna
Anconeus m.
Flexor carpi ulnaris m.
Extensor carpi ulnaris m.
Extensor digiti minimi m.
Extensor retinaculum
Extensor indicis t.
Extensor carpi ulnaris t.
5th metacarpal bone
Extensor digiti minimi t.
Extensor digitorum t.

Triceps brachii m.
Superior ulnar collateral artery
Brachioradialis m.
Extensor carpi radialis longus m.
Common extensor t.
Extensor carpi radialis brevis m.
Extensor digitorum m.
Abductor pollicis longus m.
Extensor pollicis brevis m.
Extensor carpi radialis brevis t.
Extensor carpi radialis longus t.
Extensor pollicis longus t.
Radial artery
Abductor pollicis longus t.
Anatomical snuffbox
Extensor pollicis brevis t.
Extensor pollicis longus t.

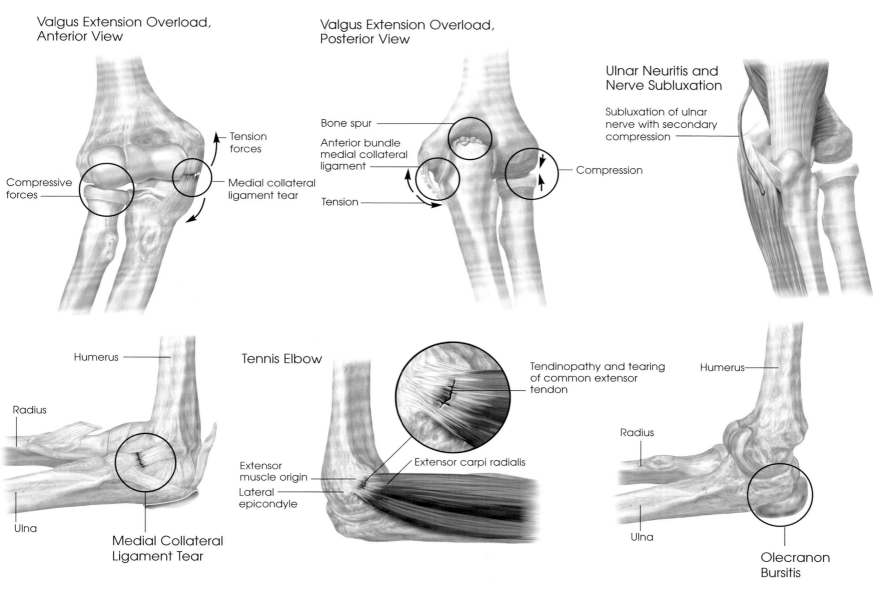

Valgus Extension Overload, Anterior View

Tension forces

Compressive forces

Medial collateral ligament tear

Valgus Extension Overload, Posterior View

Bone spur

Anterior bundle medial collateral ligament

Tension

Compression

Ulnar Neuritis and Nerve Subluxation

Subluxation of ulnar nerve with secondary compression

Humerus

Radius

Ulna

Medial Collateral Ligament Tear

Tennis Elbow

Tendinopathy and tearing of common extensor tendon

Extensor muscle origin

Lateral epicondyle

Extensor carpi radialis

Humerus

Radius

Ulna

Olecranon Bursitis

Movements

Supination

Pronation

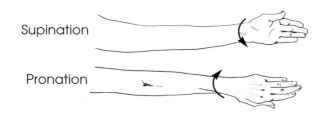

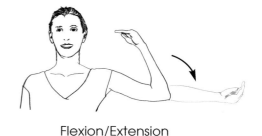

Flexion/Extension

Mechanism of Injury

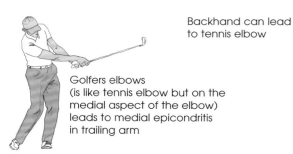

Golfers elbows (is like tennis elbow but on the medial aspect of the elbow) leads to medial epicondritis in trailing arm

Backhand can lead to tennis elbow

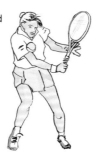

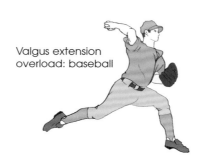

Valgus extension overload: baseball

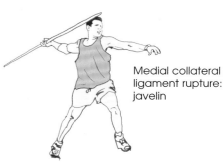

Medial collateral ligament rupture: javelin

Normal Anatomy–
Growth Plates and Ossification Sites

Distal End of Humerus

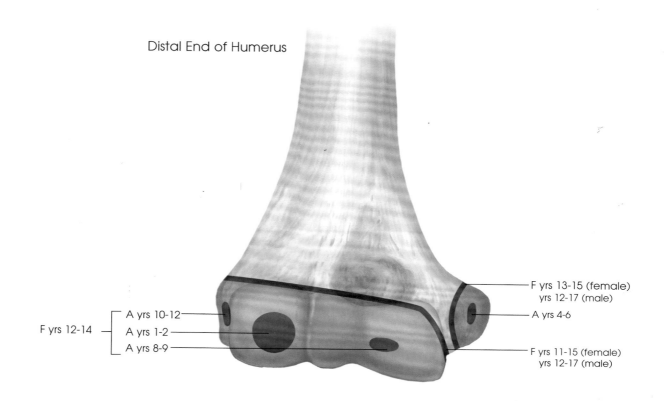

F yrs 13-15 (female)
yrs 12-17 (male)

A yrs 10-12

A yrs 4-6

F yrs 12-14   A yrs 1-2

A yrs 8-9

F yrs 11-15 (female)
yrs 12-17 (male)

Proximal End of Radius

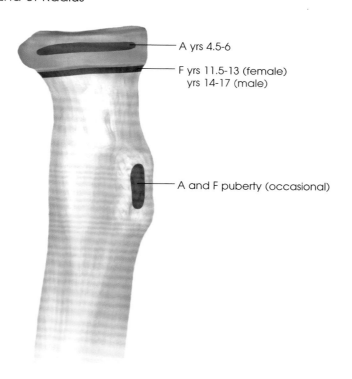

A yrs 4.5-6

F yrs 11.5-13 (female)
yrs 14-17 (male)

A and F puberty (occasional)

Proximal End of Ulna

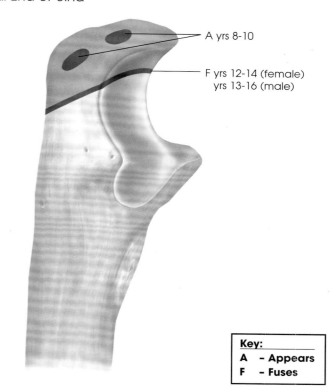

A yrs 8-10

F yrs 12-14 (female)
yrs 13-16 (male)

Key:
A – Appears
F – Fuses

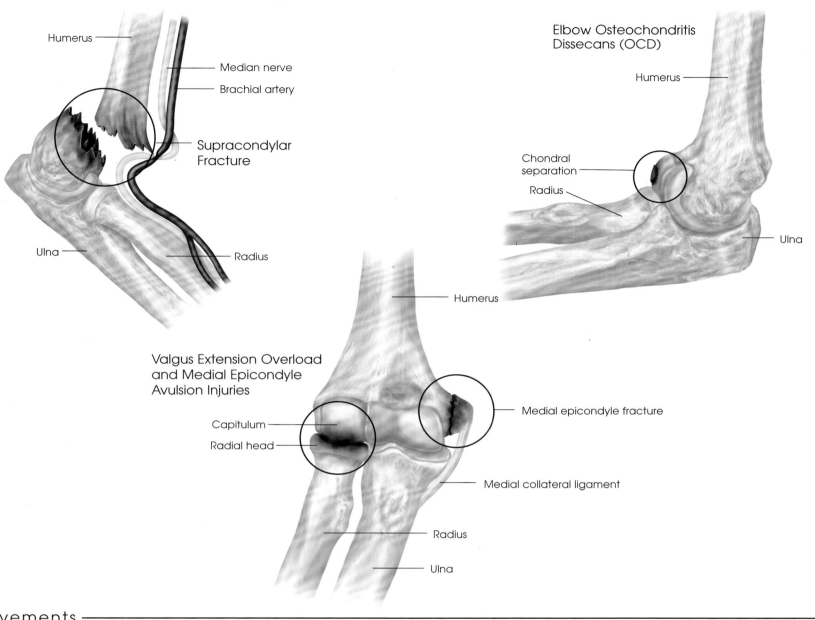

Humerus

Median nerve

Brachial artery

Supracondylar
Fracture

Ulna

Radius

Elbow Osteochondritis
Dissecans (OCD)

Humerus

Chondral
separation

Radius

Ulna

Humerus

Valgus Extension Overload
and Medial Epicondyle
Avulsion Injuries

Medial epicondyle fracture

Capitulum

Radial head

Medial collateral ligament

Radius

Ulna

Movements

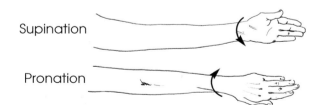

Supination

Pronation

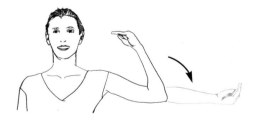

Flexion/Extension

Mechanism of Injury

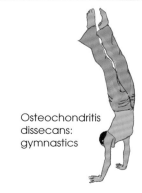

Supracondylar
fracture

Osteochondritis
dissecans:
gymnastics

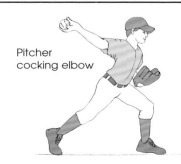

Pitcher
cocking elbow

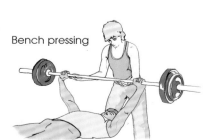

Bench pressing

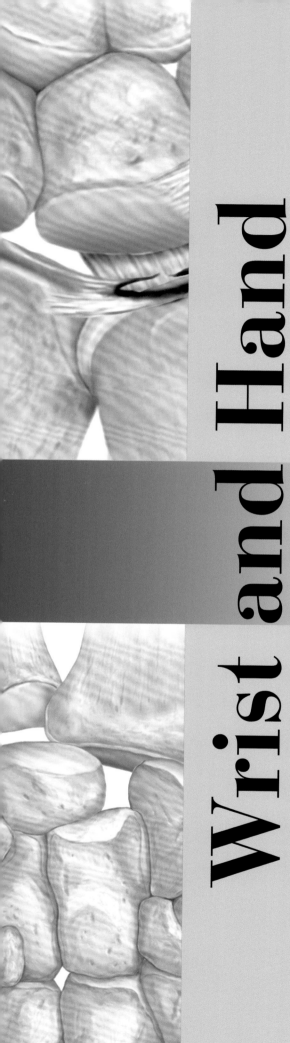

Wrist and Hand

A Complex Anatomy

The wrist and hand account for some of the most complex anatomy of the musculoskeletal system. Most sports use the hand as the key action endpoint for the athlete whether they are throwing, catching or hitting. Repetitive wrist movement caused by racquet sports is a common cause for injury in children and adults. Finger and thumb fractures as well as inflammation and arthritis are also frequent ailments.

chapter **4**

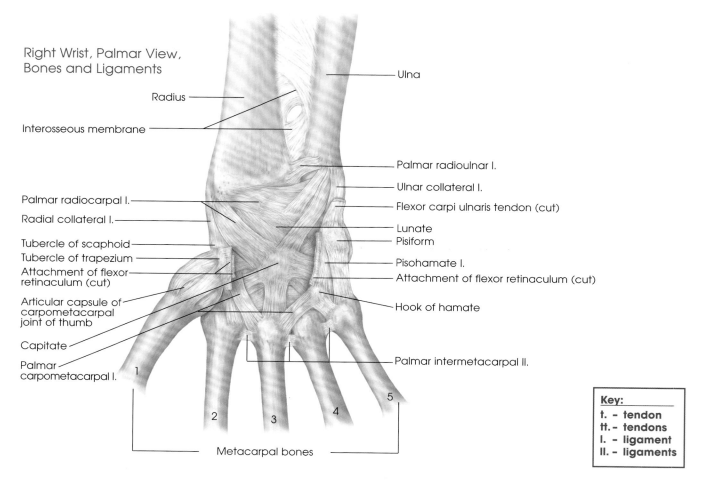

Right Wrist, Palmar View,
Bones and Ligaments

Radius —

Interosseous membrane —

Ulna

Palmar radioulnar l.

Ulnar collateral l.

Palmar radiocarpal l. —

Radial collateral l. —

Flexor carpi ulnaris tendon (cut)

Lunate

Tubercle of scaphoid —

Pisiform

Tubercle of trapezium —

Pisohamate l.

Attachment of flexor
retinaculum (cut) —

Attachment of flexor retinaculum (cut)

Articular capsule of
carpometacarpal
joint of thumb —

Hook of hamate

Capitate —

Palmar
carpometacarpal l. —

Palmar intermetacarpal ll.

1

2   3   4   5

Metacarpal bones

Key:
t. – **tendon**
tt. – **tendons**
l. – **ligament**
ll. – **ligaments**

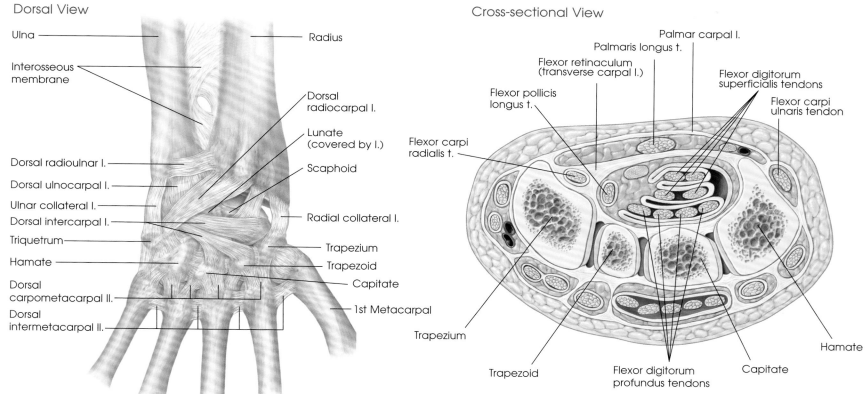

Dorsal View

Ulna —

Radius

Interosseous
membrane —

Dorsal
radiocarpal l.

Dorsal radioulnar l. —

Lunate
(covered by l.)

Dorsal ulnocarpal l. —

Scaphoid

Ulnar collateral l. —

Dorsal intercarpal l. —

Triquetrum —

Radial collateral l.

Hamate —

Trapezium

Dorsal
carpometacarpal ll. —

Trapezoid

Capitate

Dorsal
intermetacarpal ll. —

1st Metacarpal

Cross-sectional View

Palmar carpal l.

Palmaris longus t.

Flexor retinaculum
(transverse carpal l.)

Flexor digitorum
superficialis tendons

Flexor pollicis
longus t.

Flexor carpi
ulnaris tendon

Flexor carpi
radialis t.

Trapezium

Hamate

Trapezoid

Capitate

Flexor digitorum
profundus tendons

Wrist fractures

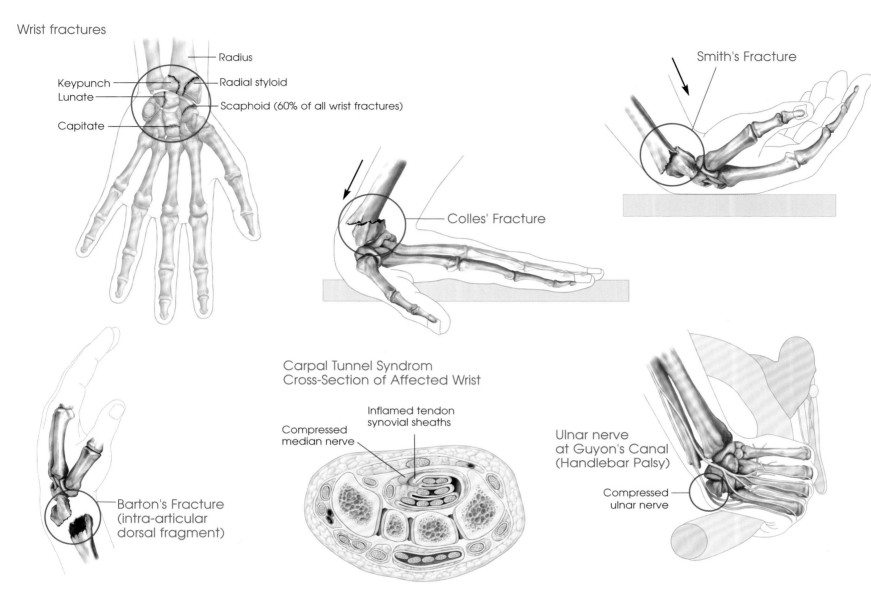

Radius

Keypunch

Radial styloid

Lunate

Scaphoid (60% of all wrist fractures)

Capitate

Smith's Fracture

Colles' Fracture

Barton's Fracture
(intra-articular
dorsal fragment)

Carpal Tunnel Syndrom
Cross-Section of Affected Wrist

Inflamed tendon
synovial sheaths

Compressed
median nerve

Ulnar nerve
at Guyon's Canal
(Handlebar Palsy)

Compressed
ulnar nerve

Movements

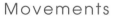

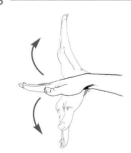

Wrist Flexion/
Extension

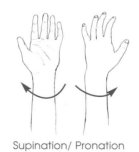

Supination/ Pronation

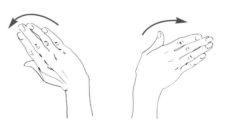

Radial Deviation/Ulnar Deviation

Mechanism of Injury

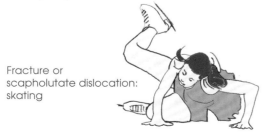

Fracture or
scapholutate dislocation:
skating

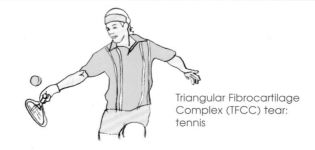

Triangular Fibrocartilage
Complex (TFCC) tear:
tennis

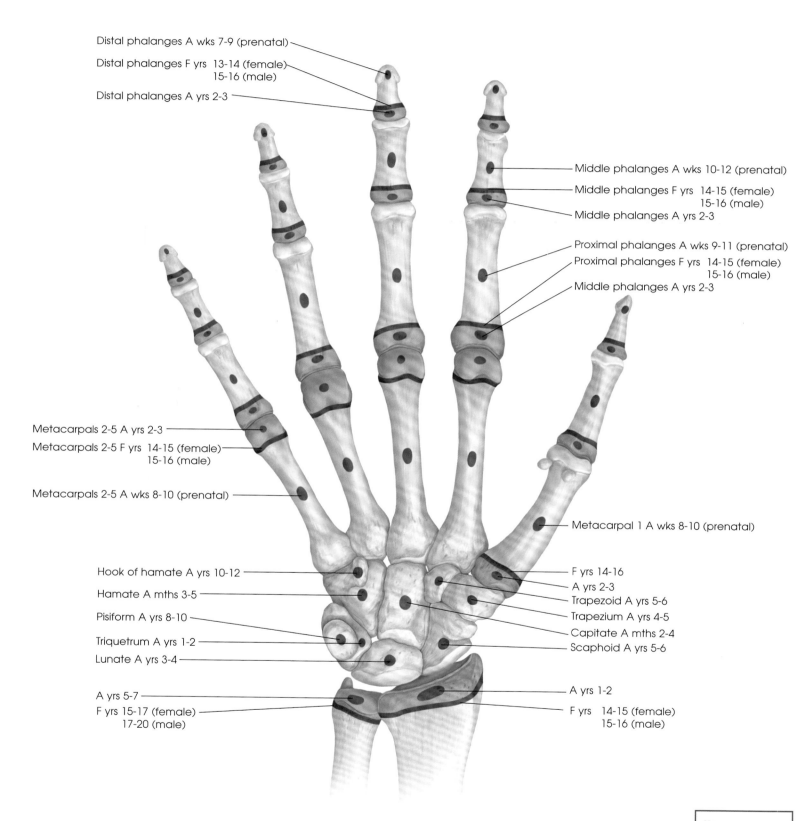

Distal phalanges A wks 7-9 (prenatal)

Distal phalanges F yrs 13-14 (female)
15-16 (male)

Distal phalanges A yrs 2-3

Middle phalanges A wks 10-12 (prenatal)

Middle phalanges F yrs 14-15 (female)
15-16 (male)

Middle phalanges A yrs 2-3

Proximal phalanges A wks 9-11 (prenatal)

Proximal phalanges F yrs 14-15 (female)
15-16 (male)

Middle phalanges A yrs 2-3

Metacarpals 2-5 A yrs 2-3

Metacarpals 2-5 F yrs 14-15 (female)
15-16 (male)

Metacarpals 2-5 A wks 8-10 (prenatal)

Metacarpal 1 A wks 8-10 (prenatal)

Hook of hamate A yrs 10-12

Hamate A mths 3-5

Pisiform A yrs 8-10

Triquetrum A yrs 1-2

Lunate A yrs 3-4

F yrs 14-16

A yrs 2-3

Trapezoid A yrs 5-6

Trapezium A yrs 4-5

Capitate A mths 2-4

Scaphoid A yrs 5-6

A yrs 5-7

F yrs 15-17 (female)
17-20 (male)

A yrs 1-2

F yrs 14-15 (female)
15-16 (male)

Key:
A – **Appears**
F – **Fuses**

Triangular Fibrocartilage Complex
(TFCC) Tear

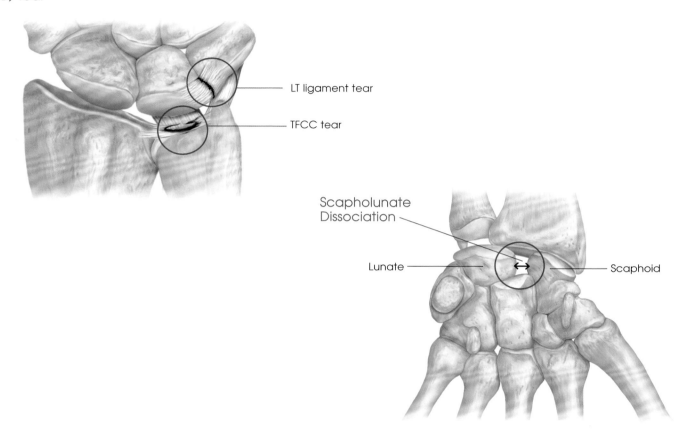

—— LT ligament tear

—— TFCC tear

Scapholunate
Dissociation

Lunate ——

Scaphoid

Movements

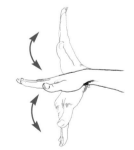

Wrist Flexion
Extension

Supination/Pronation

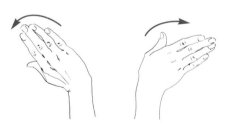

Radial Deviation/Ulnar Deviation

Mechanism of Injury

Triangular Fibrocartilage
Complex (TFCC) Tear:
baseball

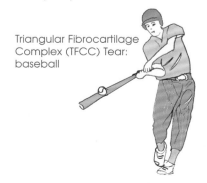

Dorsal wrist impingement
distal radius physeal injury:
gymnastics

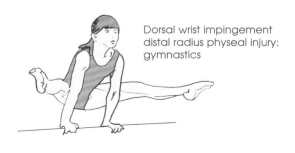

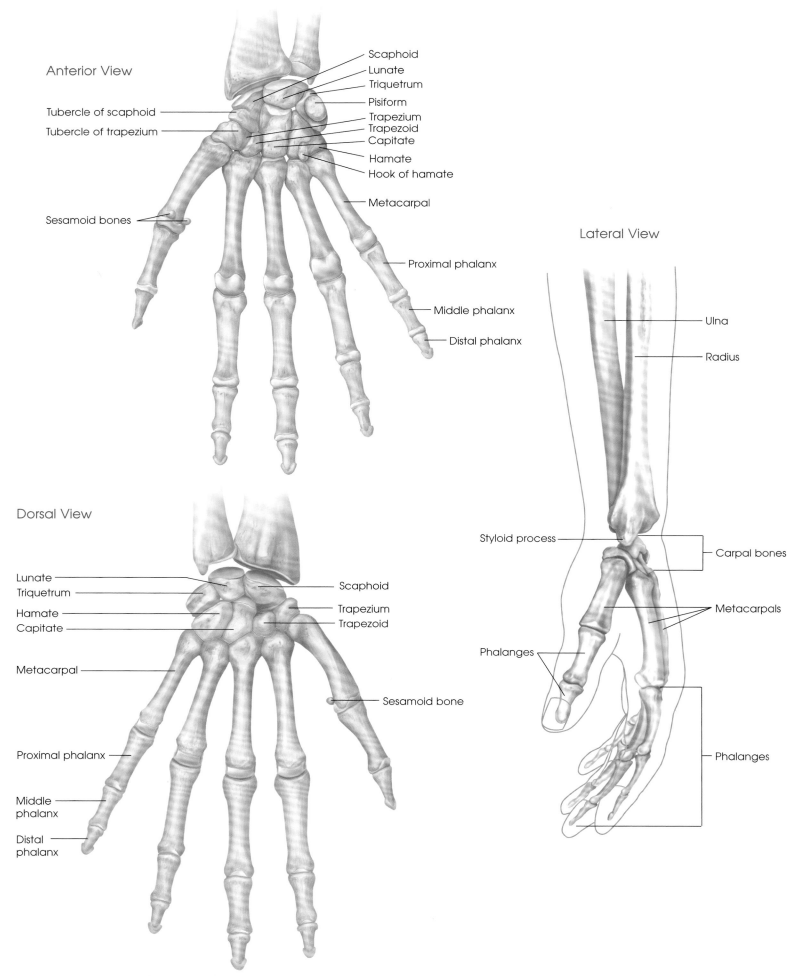

Anterior View

Scaphoid
Lunate
Triquetrum
Pisiform
Trapezium
Trapezoid
Capitate
Hamate
Hook of hamate

Tubercle of scaphoid
Tubercle of trapezium

Sesamoid bones

Metacarpal

Proximal phalanx

Middle phalanx

Distal phalanx

Lateral View

Ulna

Radius

Dorsal View

Lunate
Triquetrum
Hamate
Capitate

Scaphoid

Trapezium
Trapezoid

Metacarpal

Sesamoid bone

Proximal phalanx

Middle phalanx

Distal phalanx

Styloid process

Carpal bones

Metacarpals

Phalanges

Phalanges

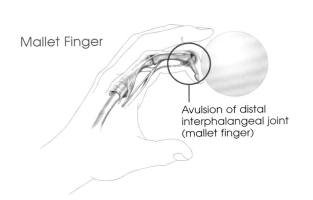

Mallet Finger

Avulsion of distal
interphalangeal joint
(mallet finger)

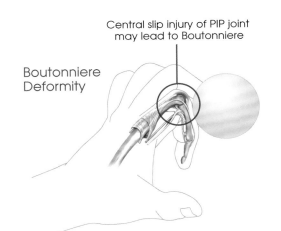

Central slip injury of PIP joint
may lead to Boutonniere

Boutonniere
Deformity

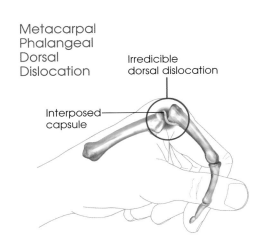

Metacarpal
Phalangeal
Dorsal
Dislocation

Irredicible
dorsal dislocation

Interposed
capsule

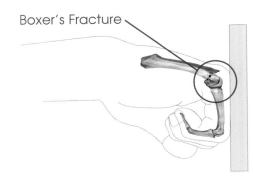

Boxer's Fracture

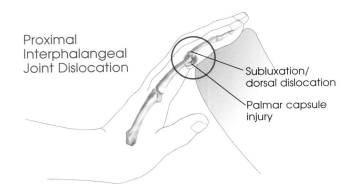

Proximal
Interphalangeal
Joint Dislocation

Subluxation/
dorsal dislocation

Palmar capsule
injury

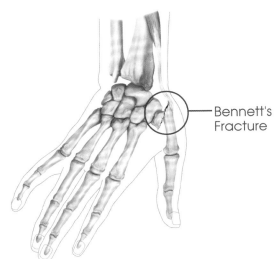

Bennett's
Fracture

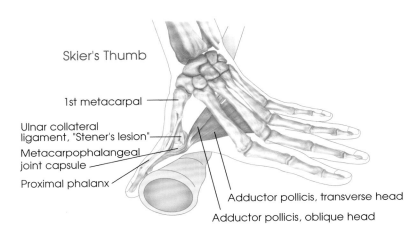

Skier's Thumb

1st metacarpal

Ulnar collateral
ligament, "Stener's lesion"

Metacarpophalangeal
joint capsule

Proximal phalanx

Adductor pollicis, transverse head

Adductor pollicis, oblique head

Movements ——

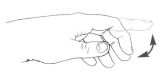

Finger extension/ Finger flexion

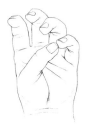

Thumb opposition

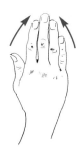

Finger adduction

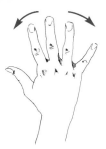

Finger abduction

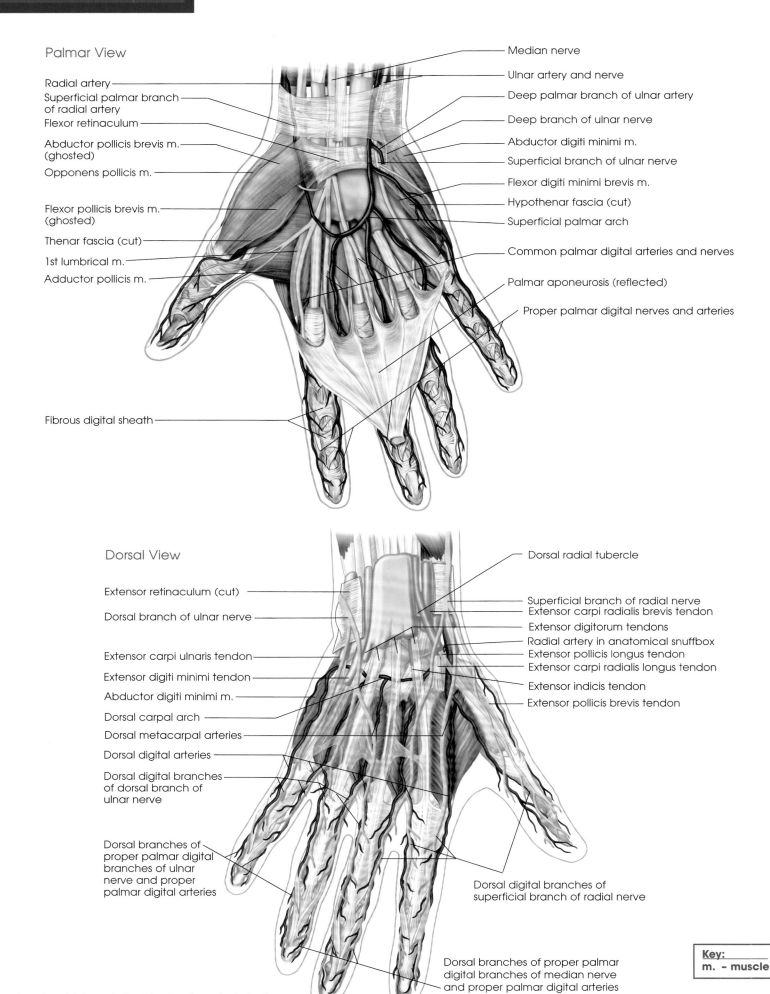

Palmar View

Radial artery

Superficial palmar branch of radial artery

Flexor retinaculum

Abductor pollicis brevis m. (ghosted)

Opponens pollicis m.

Flexor pollicis brevis m. (ghosted)

Thenar fascia (cut)

1st lumbrical m.

Adductor pollicis m.

Fibrous digital sheath

Median nerve

Ulnar artery and nerve

Deep palmar branch of ulnar artery

Deep branch of ulnar nerve

Abductor digiti minimi m.

Superficial branch of ulnar nerve

Flexor digiti minimi brevis m.

Hypothenar fascia (cut)

Superficial palmar arch

Common palmar digital arteries and nerves

Palmar aponeurosis (reflected)

Proper palmar digital nerves and arteries

Dorsal View

Extensor retinaculum (cut)

Dorsal branch of ulnar nerve

Extensor carpi ulnaris tendon

Extensor digiti minimi tendon

Abductor digiti minimi m.

Dorsal carpal arch

Dorsal metacarpal arteries

Dorsal digital arteries

Dorsal digital branches of dorsal branch of ulnar nerve

Dorsal branches of proper palmar digital branches of ulnar nerve and proper palmar digital arteries

Dorsal radial tubercle

Superficial branch of radial nerve

Extensor carpi radialis brevis tendon

Extensor digitorum tendons

Radial artery in anatomical snuffbox

Extensor pollicis longus tendon

Extensor carpi radialis longus tendon

Extensor indicis tendon

Extensor pollicis brevis tendon

Dorsal digital branches of superficial branch of radial nerve

Dorsal branches of proper palmar digital branches of median nerve and proper palmar digital arteries

Key:
m. – muscle

Inflammation and Arthritis

Wrist and Hand

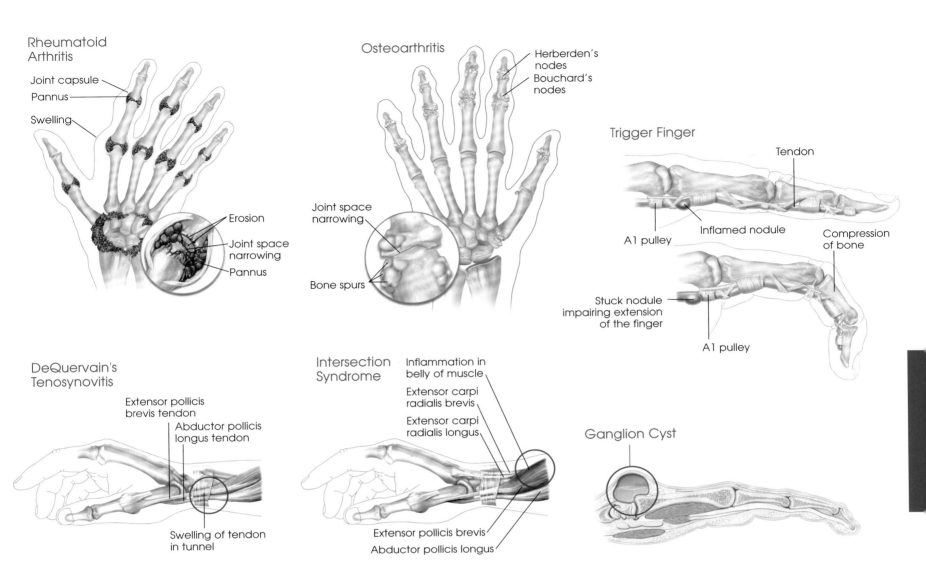

Rheumatoid Arthritis

- Joint capsule
- Pannus
- Swelling
- Erosion
- Joint space narrowing
- Pannus

Osteoarthritis

- Herberden's nodes
- Bouchard's nodes
- Joint space narrowing
- Bone spurs

Trigger Finger

- Tendon
- A1 pulley
- Inflamed nodule
- Compression of bone
- Stuck nodule impairing extension of the finger
- A1 pulley

DeQuervain's Tenosynovitis

- Extensor pollicis brevis tendon
- Abductor pollicis longus tendon
- Swelling of tendon in tunnel

Intersection Syndrome

- Inflammation in belly of muscle
- Extensor carpi radialis brevis
- Extensor carpi radialis longus
- Extensor pollicis brevis
- Abductor pollicis longus

Ganglion Cyst

Movements

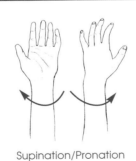

Wrist Flexion Extension

Supination/Pronation

Radial Deviation/Ulnar Deviation

Mechanism of Injury

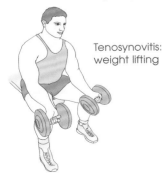

Tenosynovitis: weight lifting

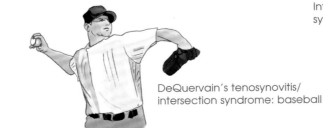

DeQuervain's tenosynovitis/ intersection syndrome: baseball

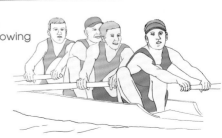

Intersection syndrome: rowing

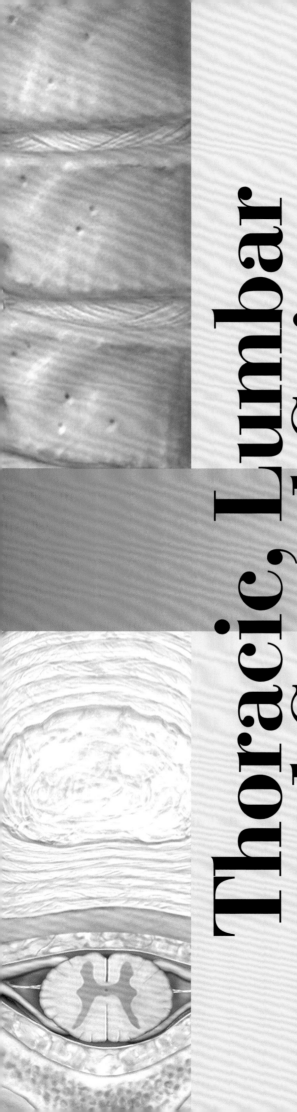

Thoracic, Lumbar and Sacral Spine

The Foundation

The core of the musculoskeletal system is the cervical, thoracic, lumbar and sacral spine. This central structure serves as the foundation for force development as well as an anchor for the appendicular skeleton. Sports that require repetitive extension, rotational or power lifting such as gymnastics, golf, football and weight lifting, increase the risk of stress fractures of the lumbar spine. Abnormalities and injuries in the spine may be related to injuries along the appendicular skeleton.

chapter

5

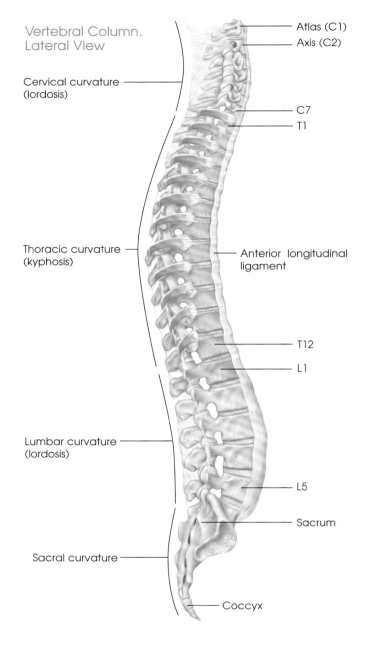

Vertebral Column,
Lateral View

Cervical curvature
(lordosis)

Atlas (C1)

Axis (C2)

C7

T1

Thoracic curvature
(kyphosis)

Anterior longitudinal
ligament

T12

L1

Lumbar curvature
(lordosis)

L5

Sacrum

Sacral curvature

Coccyx

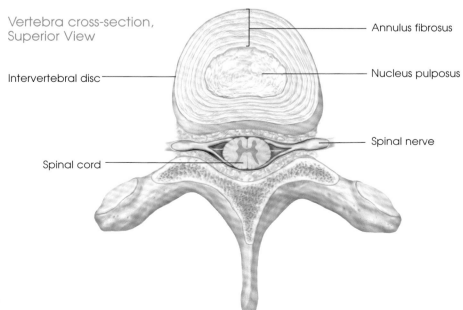

Vertebra cross-section,
Superior View

Annulus fibrosus

Nucleus pulposus

Intervertebral disc

Spinal nerve

Spinal cord

Thoracic, Lumbar and Sacral Spine Problems

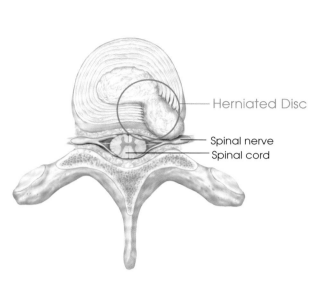

Herniated Disc

Spinal nerve
Spinal cord

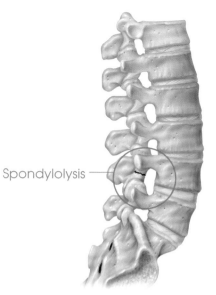

Spondylolysis

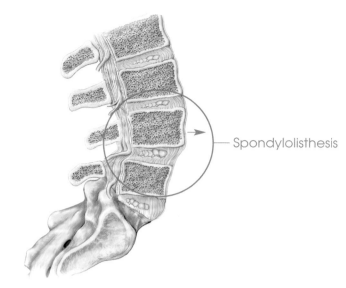

Spondylolisthesis

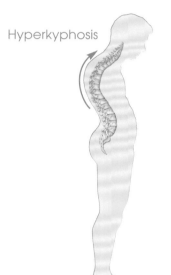

Hyperkyphosis

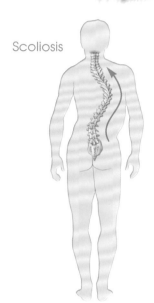

Scoliosis

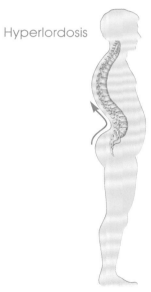

Hyperlordosis

Movements

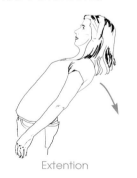

Extention

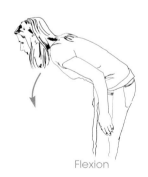

Flexion

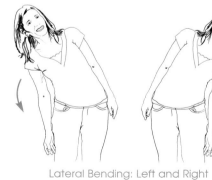

Lateral Bending: Left and Right

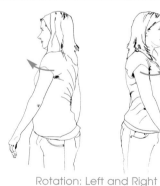
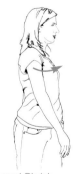

Rotation: Left and Right

Mechanism of Injury

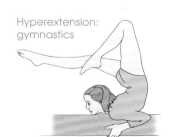

Hyperextension: gymnastics

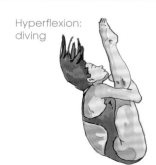

Hyperflexion: diving

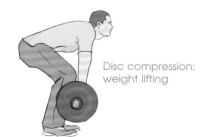

Disc compression: weight lifting

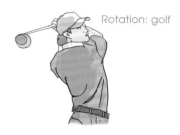

Rotation: golf

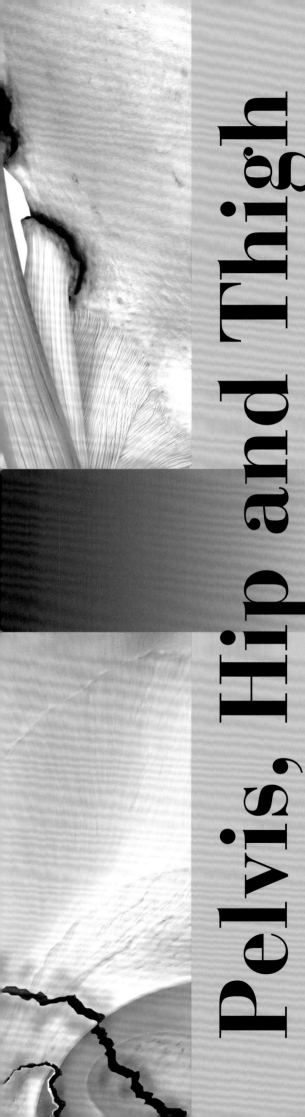

Pelvis, Hip and Thigh

The Basis for Motion

The pelvis and hip provide a basis for motion, gait and transfer of forces between the core and lower extremity. Runners and cyclists, sports with increased demands of hip flexibility such as soccer, and those that require extremes of motion such as gymnastics, have an increased risk of hip fracture, dislocation or soft tissue injuries such as ligament tears.

chapter **6**

Pelvis, Anterior View

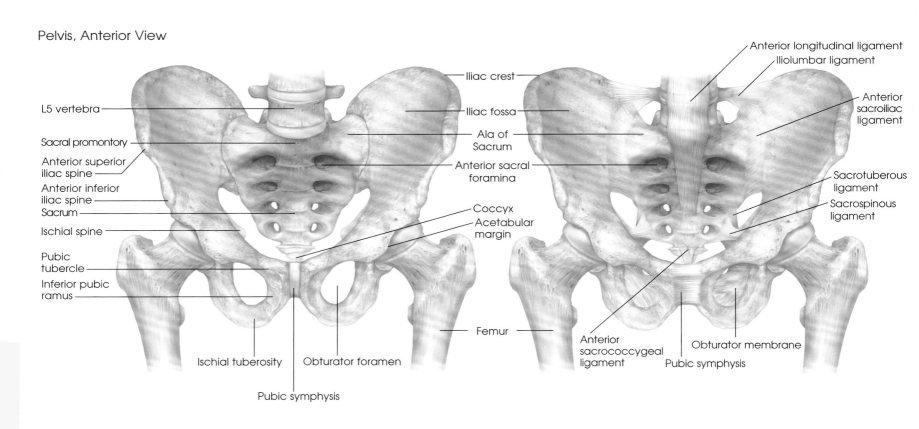

L5 vertebra

Sacral promontory

Anterior superior iliac spine

Anterior inferior iliac spine

Sacrum

Ischial spine

Pubic tubercle

Inferior pubic ramus

Iliac crest

Iliac fossa

Ala of Sacrum

Anterior sacral foramina

Coccyx

Acetabular margin

Ischial tuberosity

Obturator foramen

Femur

Pubic symphysis

Anterior longitudinal ligament

Iliolumbar ligament

Anterior sacroiliac ligament

Sacrotuberous ligament

Sacrospinous ligament

Anterior sacrococcygeal ligament

Obturator membrane

Pubic symphysis

Key:
A – **Appears**
F – **Fuses**
m. – **muscle**

Muscles and Nerves

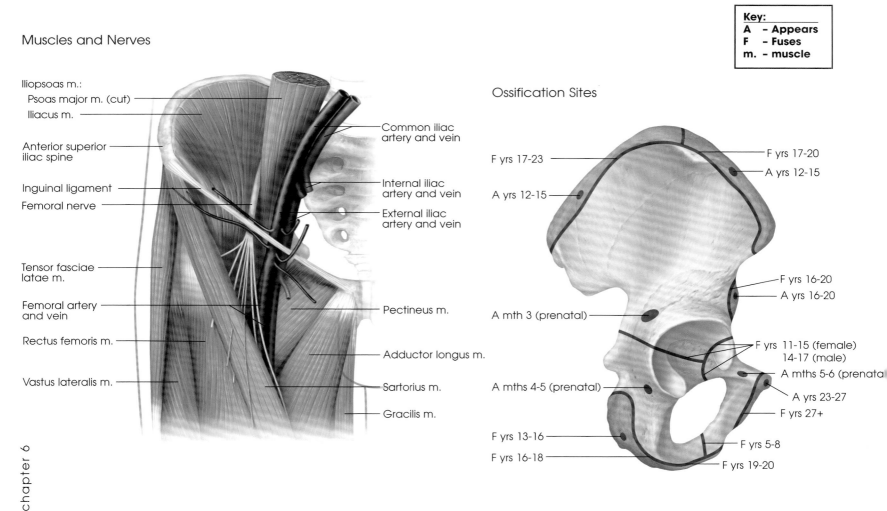

Iliopsoas m.:
  Psoas major m. (cut)
  Iliacus m.

Anterior superior iliac spine

Inguinal ligament

Femoral nerve

Tensor fasciae latae m.

Femoral artery and vein

Rectus femoris m.

Vastus lateralis m.

Common iliac artery and vein

Internal iliac artery and vein

External iliac artery and vein

Pectineus m.

Adductor longus m.

Sartorius m.

Gracilis m.

Ossification Sites

F yrs 17-23

A yrs 12-15

A mth 3 (prenatal)

A mths 4-5 (prenatal)

F yrs 13-16

F yrs 16-18

F yrs 17-20

A yrs 12-15

F yrs 16-20

A yrs 16-20

F yrs 11-15 (female)
14-17 (male)

A mths 5-6 (prenatal)

A yrs 23-27

F yrs 27+

F yrs 5-8

F yrs 19-20

Injuries of the Pelvis and Acetabulum (children and adults)

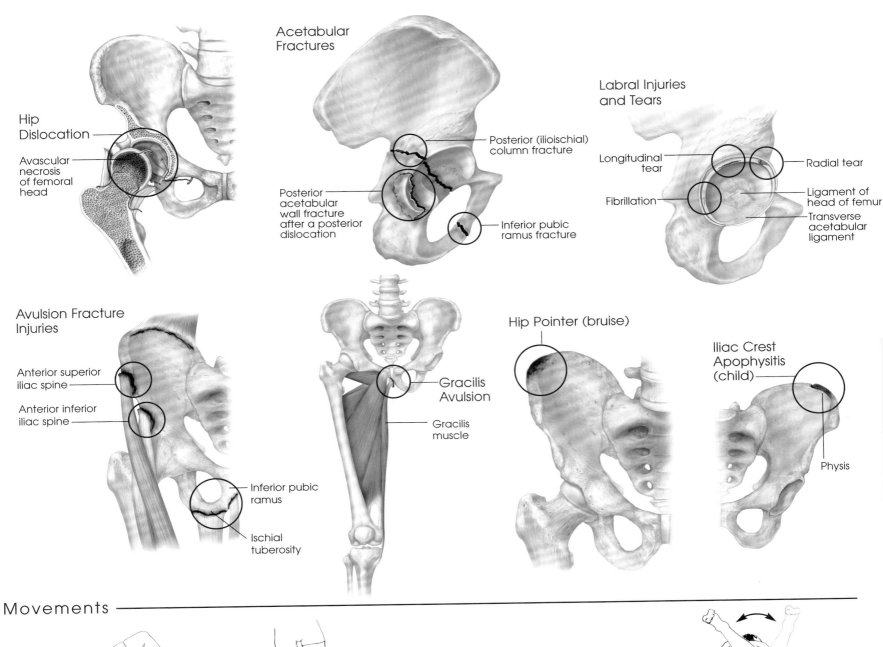

Hip Dislocation

Avascular necrosis of femoral head

Acetabular Fractures

Posterior (ilioischial) column fracture

Posterior acetabular wall fracture after a posterior dislocation

Inferior pubic ramus fracture

Labral Injuries and Tears

Longitudinal tear

Radial tear

Fibrillation

Ligament of head of femur

Transverse acetabular ligament

Avulsion Fracture Injuries

Anterior superior iliac spine

Anterior inferior iliac spine

Inferior pubic ramus

Ischial tuberosity

Gracilis Avulsion

Gracilis muscle

Hip Pointer (bruise)

Iliac Crest Apophysitis (child)

Physis

Movements

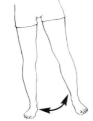
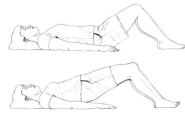

Pelvic tilt

Abduction/Adduction

Flexion/Extension

Internal External rotation

Mechanism of Injury

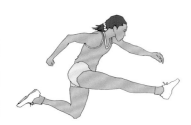

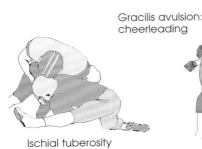

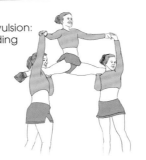

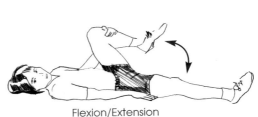

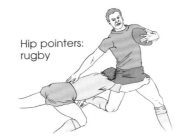

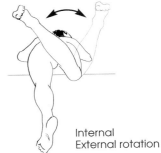

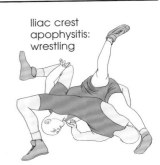

Anterior superior iliac spine (ASIS) avulsion: hurdling

Ischial tuberosity avulsion: football

Gracilis avulsion: cheerleading

Hip pointers: rugby

Iliac crest apophysitis: wrestling

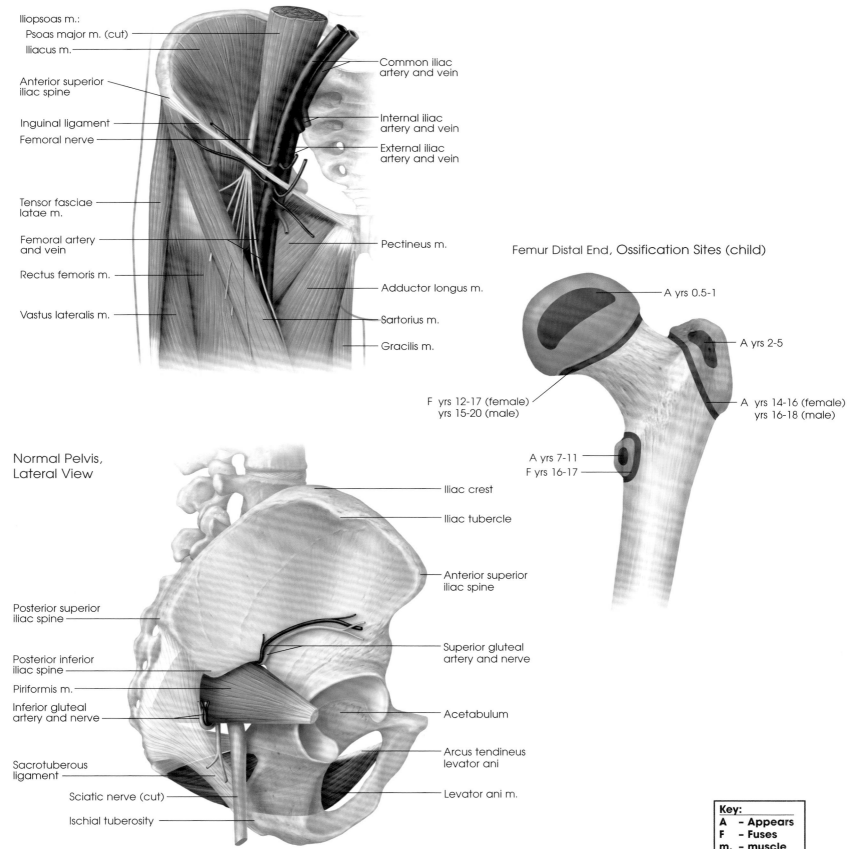

Pelvis and Anterior Thigh,
Anterior View with Muscles and Nerves

Iliopsoas m.:
Psoas major m. (cut)
Iliacus m.
Anterior superior iliac spine
Inguinal ligament
Femoral nerve
Tensor fasciae latae m.
Femoral artery and vein
Rectus femoris m.
Vastus lateralis m.

Common iliac artery and vein
Internal iliac artery and vein
External iliac artery and vein
Pectineus m.
Adductor longus m.
Sartorius m.
Gracilis m.

Femur Distal End, Ossification Sites (child)

A yrs 0.5-1
A yrs 2-5
F yrs 12-17 (female) yrs 15-20 (male)
A yrs 14-16 (female) yrs 16-18 (male)
A yrs 7-11
F yrs 16-17

Normal Pelvis,
Lateral View

Posterior superior iliac spine
Posterior inferior iliac spine
Piriformis m.
Inferior gluteal artery and nerve
Sacrotuberous ligament
Sciatic nerve (cut)
Ischial tuberosity

Iliac crest
Iliac tubercle
Anterior superior iliac spine
Superior gluteal artery and nerve
Acetabulum
Arcus tendineus levator ani
Levator ani m.

Key:
A – **Appears**
F – **Fuses**
m. – **muscle**

Injuries of the Proximal Femur
(children and adults)

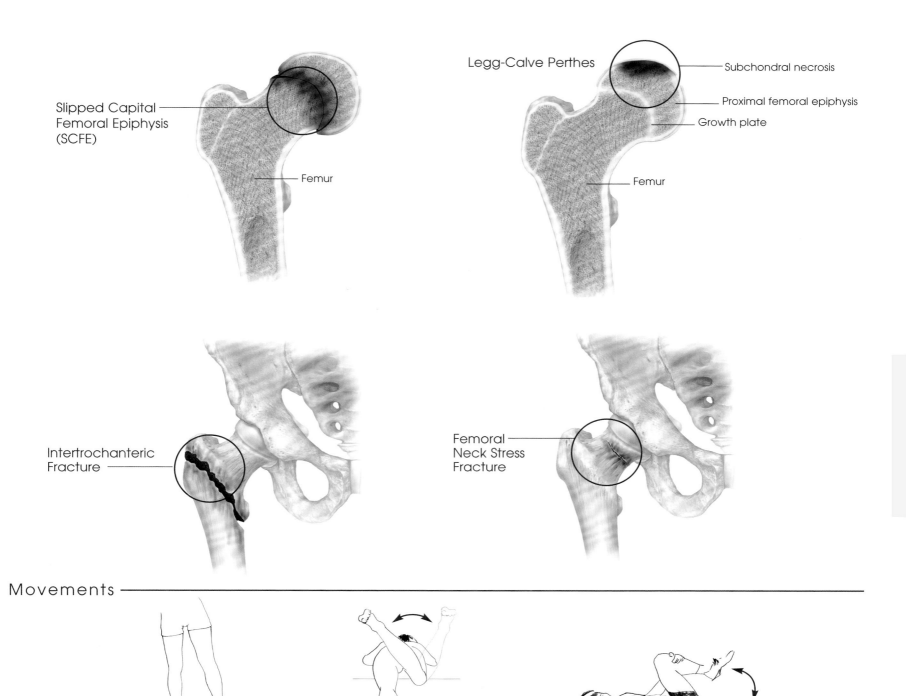

Slipped Capital Femoral Epiphysis (SCFE)

Femur

Legg-Calve Perthes

Subchondral necrosis

Proximal femoral epiphysis

Growth plate

Femur

Intertrochanteric Fracture

Femoral Neck Stress Fracture

Movements

Abduction/Adduction

Hip Join Rotation

Flexion/Extension

Mechanism of Injury

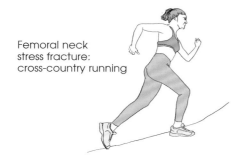

Femoral neck stress fracture: cross-country running

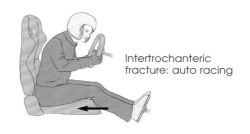

Intertrochanteric fracture: auto racing

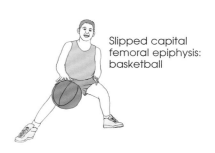

Slipped capital femoral epiphysis: basketball

Anterior View

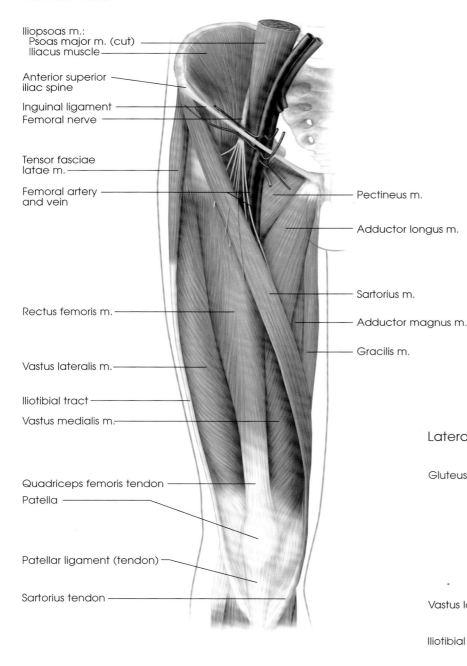

Iliopsoas m.:
  Psoas major m. (cut)
  Iliacus muscle

Anterior superior
iliac spine

Inguinal ligament
Femoral nerve

Tensor fasciae
latae m.

Femoral artery
and vein

Rectus femoris m.

Vastus lateralis m.

Iliotibial tract

Vastus medialis m.

Quadriceps femoris tendon

Patella

Patellar ligament (tendon)

Sartorius tendon

Pectineus m.

Adductor longus m.

Sartorius m.

Adductor magnus m.

Gracilis m.

Lateral View

Gluteus maximus m.

Vastus lateralis m.

Iliotibial tract

Biceps femoris m.
  Long head
  Short head

Semimembranosus m.

Sartorius m.

Tensor fasciae
latae m.

Rectus femoris m

Key:
m. – muscle

Hip and Thigh Soft Tissue Problems

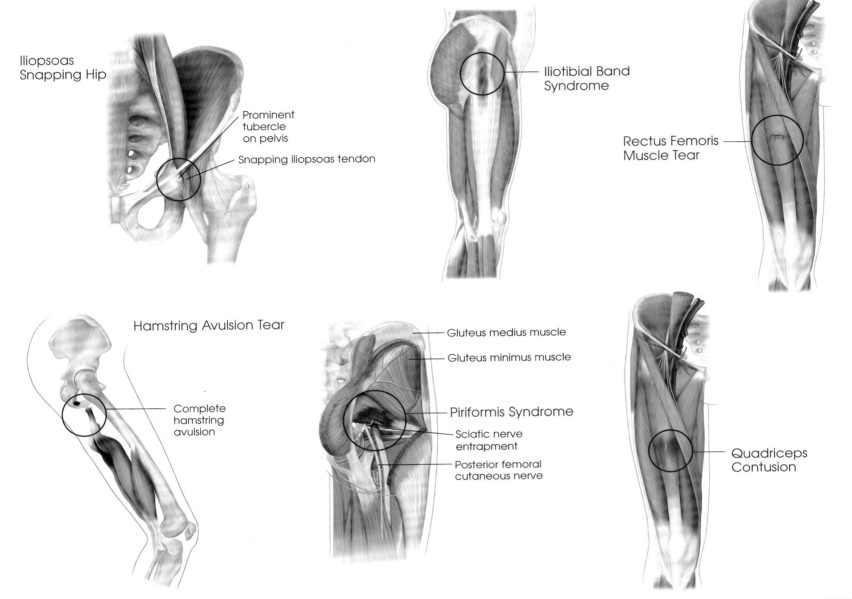

Iliopsoas
Snapping Hip

Prominent
tubercle
on pelvis

Snapping iliopsoas tendon

Iliotibial Band
Syndrome

Rectus Femoris
Muscle Tear

Hamstring Avulsion Tear

Complete
hamstring
avulsion

Gluteus medius muscle

Gluteus minimus muscle

Piriformis Syndrome

Sciatic nerve
entrapment

Posterior femoral
cutaneous nerve

Quadriceps
Contusion

Movements

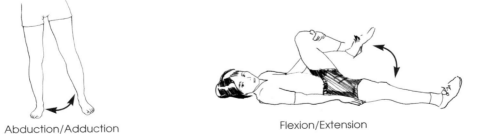

Abduction/Adduction

Flexion/Extension

Mechanism of Injury

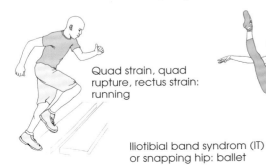

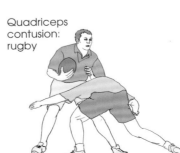

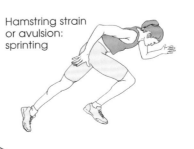

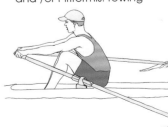

Quad strain, quad
rupture, rectus strain:
running

Iliotibial band syndrom (IT)
or snapping hip: ballet

Quadriceps
contusion:
rugby

Hamstring strain
or avulsion:
sprinting

Sciatic nerve entrapment
and /or Piriformis: rowing

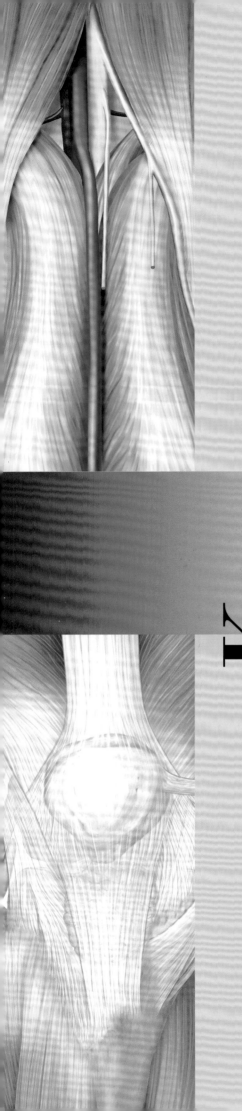

Knee

The Common Target

Because of the knee's complexity, the number of structures involved and its relatively high risk of injury, it is one of the most studied joints in sports. A knee injury can affect any of the ligaments, tendons or fluid-filled sacs (bursae) that surround the knee joint as well as the bones, cartilage and ligaments that form the joint itself.

chapter **7**

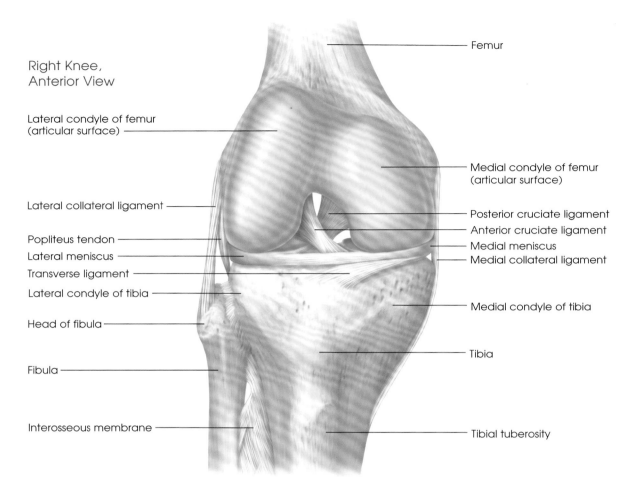

Right Knee,
Anterior View

Femur

Lateral condyle of femur
(articular surface)

Medial condyle of femur
(articular surface)

Lateral collateral ligament

Posterior cruciate ligament

Anterior cruciate ligament

Popliteus tendon

Medial meniscus

Lateral meniscus

Medial collateral ligament

Transverse ligament

Lateral condyle of tibia

Medial condyle of tibia

Head of fibula

Fibula

Tibia

Interosseous membrane

Tibial tuberosity

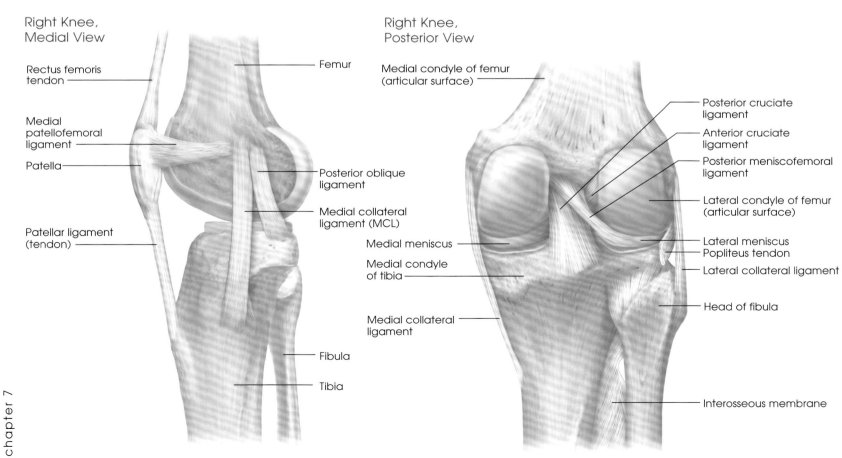

Right Knee,
Medial View

Rectus femoris
tendon

Femur

Medial
patellofemoral
ligament

Patella

Posterior oblique
ligament

Patellar ligament
(tendon)

Medial collateral
ligament (MCL)

Fibula

Tibia

Right Knee,
Posterior View

Medial condyle of femur
(articular surface)

Posterior cruciate
ligament

Anterior cruciate
ligament

Posterior meniscofemoral
ligament

Lateral condyle of femur
(articular surface)

Medial meniscus

Lateral meniscus

Medial condyle
of tibia

Popliteus tendon

Lateral collateral ligament

Medial collateral
ligament

Head of fibula

Interosseous membrane

Ligament Injuries

Bone Avulsion

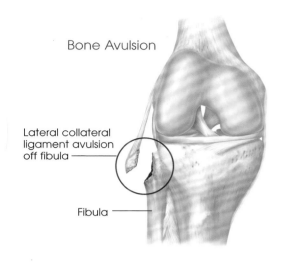

Lateral collateral ligament avulsion off fibula

Fibula

LCL Injury

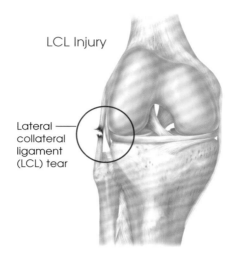

Lateral collateral ligament (LCL) tear

MCL Injury

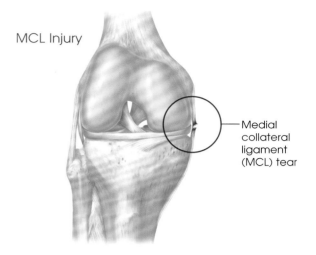

Medial collateral ligament (MCL) tear

ACL Injury

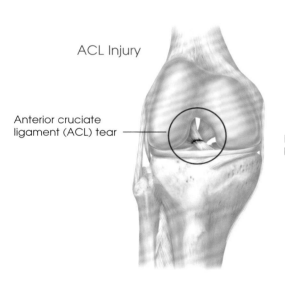

Anterior cruciate ligament (ACL) tear

PCL Injury

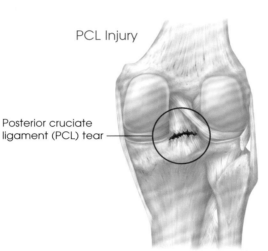

Posterior cruciate ligament (PCL) tear

Anterior Knee Dislocation

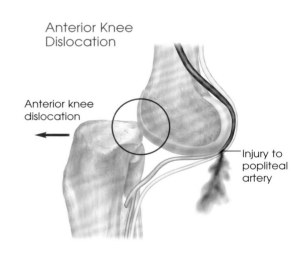

Anterior knee dislocation

Injury to popliteal artery

Movements

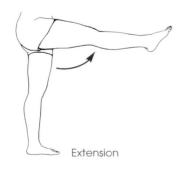

Extension

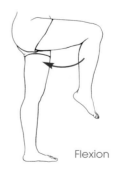

Flexion

Mechanism of Injury

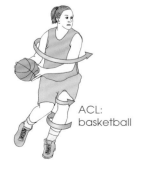

ACL: basketball

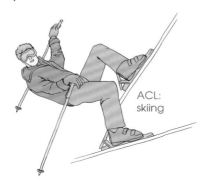

ACL: skiing

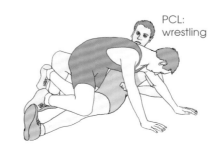

PCL: wrestling

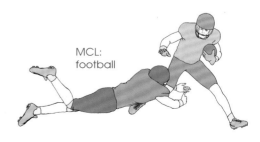

MCL: football

Right Knee Superior View

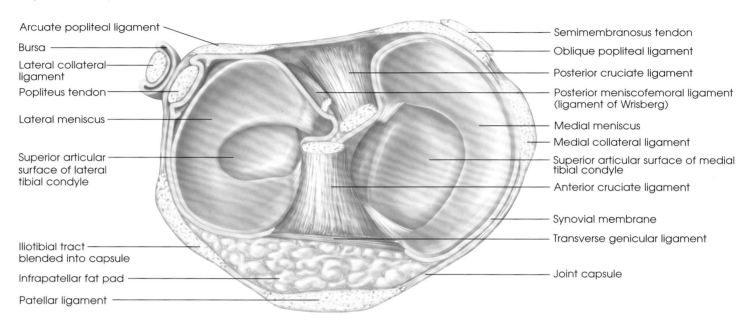

Arcuate popliteal ligament

Bursa

Lateral collateral ligament

Popliteus tendon

Lateral meniscus

Superior articular surface of lateral tibial condyle

Iliotibial tract blended into capsule

Infrapatellar fat pad

Patellar ligament

Semimembranosus tendon

Oblique popliteal ligament

Posterior cruciate ligament

Posterior meniscofemoral ligament (ligament of Wrisberg)

Medial meniscus

Medial collateral ligament

Superior articular surface of medial tibial condyle

Anterior cruciate ligament

Synovial membrane

Transverse genicular ligament

Joint capsule

Right Knee Anterior View

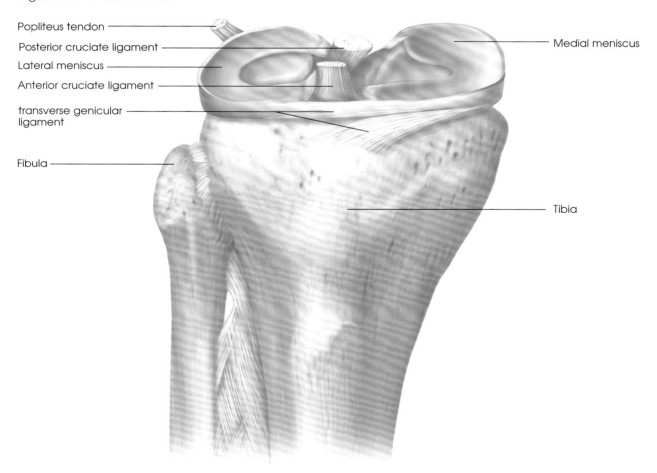

Popliteus tendon

Posterior cruciate ligament

Lateral meniscus

Anterior cruciate ligament

transverse genicular ligament

Fibula

Medial meniscus

Tibia

Meniscus Tears

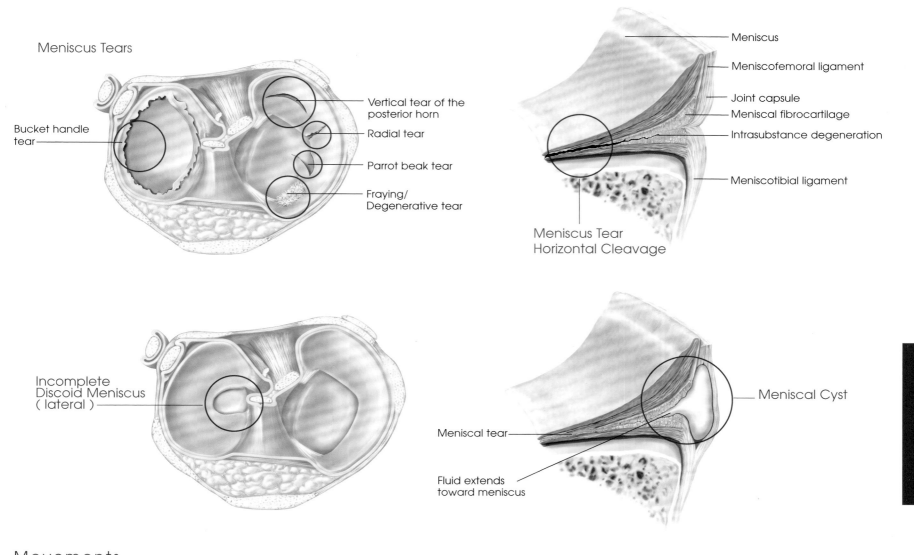

Meniscus Tears

Bucket handle tear

Vertical tear of the posterior horn

Radial tear

Parrot beak tear

Fraying/Degenerative tear

Meniscus

Meniscofemoral ligament

Joint capsule

Meniscal fibrocartilage

Intrasubstance degeneration

Meniscotibial ligament

Meniscus Tear Horizontal Cleavage

Incomplete Discoid Meniscus (lateral)

Meniscal Cyst

Meniscal tear

Fluid extends toward meniscus

Movements

Extension

Flexion

Mechanism of Injury

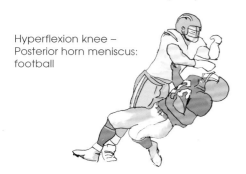

Hyperflexion knee – Posterior horn meniscus: football

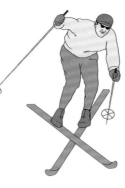

Knee twist, ACL, meniscus: gymnastics

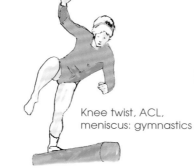

Axial Load, meniscus injury: skier landing on his extended leg

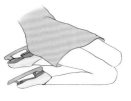

Hyperflexion, meniscus tear: skating

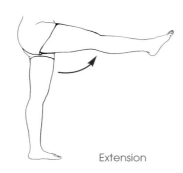
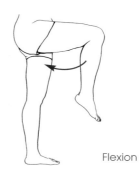

Anterior View

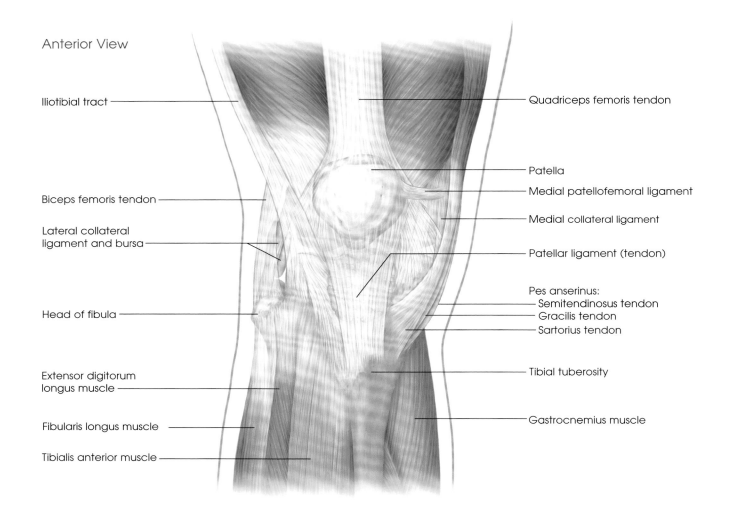

Iliotibial tract

Biceps femoris tendon

Lateral collateral ligament and bursa

Head of fibula

Extensor digitorum longus muscle

Fibularis longus muscle

Tibialis anterior muscle

Quadriceps femoris tendon

Patella

Medial patellofemoral ligament

Medial collateral ligament

Patellar ligament (tendon)

Pes anserinus:
Semitendinosus tendon
Gracilis tendon
Sartorius tendon

Tibial tuberosity

Gastrocnemius muscle

Sagittal Cross-Section

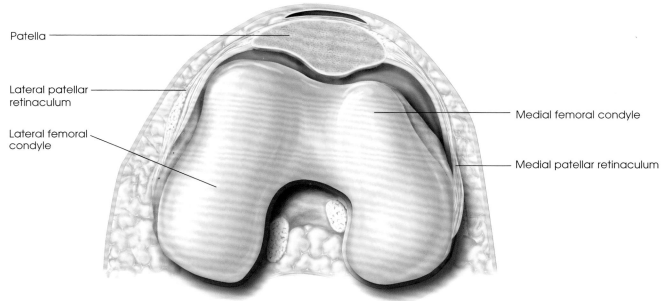

Patella

Lateral patellar retinaculum

Lateral femoral condyle

Medial femoral condyle

Medial patellar retinaculum

Extensor Mechanism Problems (adult)

Patellar Dislocation

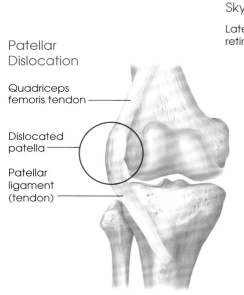

- Quadriceps femoris tendon
- Dislocated patella
- Patellar ligament (tendon)

Patellar Dislocation, Skyline View

Normal
- Lateral patellar retinaculum
- Patella
- Medial patellofemoral ligament
- Femur

Subluxation
- Medial patellofemoral ligament (stretched)

Dislocation
- Medial patellofemoral ligament (torn)

Patellar Tendinopathy

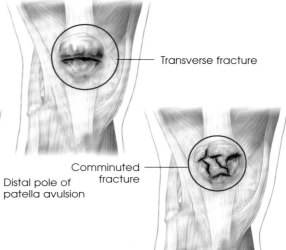

- Quadriceps femoris tendon
- Patella
- Patellar tendon (ligament)
- Tendinopathy at:
  - Distal quadriceps femoris tendon
  - Distal pole of patella
  - Tibial tuberosity

Quadriceps Tendon Rupture

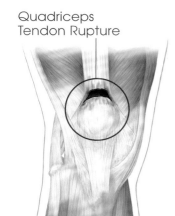

Patellar Tendon Rupture

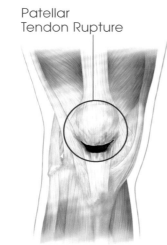

Patellar Fractures

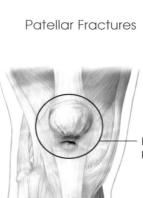

- Distal pole of patella avulsion
- Transverse fracture
- Comminuted fracture

Movements

- Extension
- Flexion

Mechanism of Injury

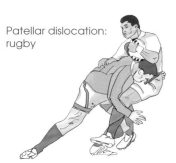

Patellar dislocation: rugby

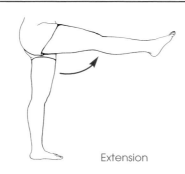

Jumper's knee: volleyball

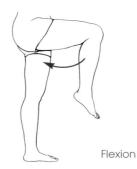

Patellar fractures: football

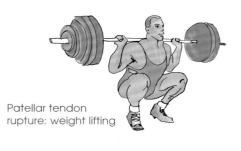

Patellar tendon rupture: weight lifting

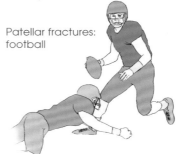

Normal Anatomy–
Growth Plates and Ossification Sites

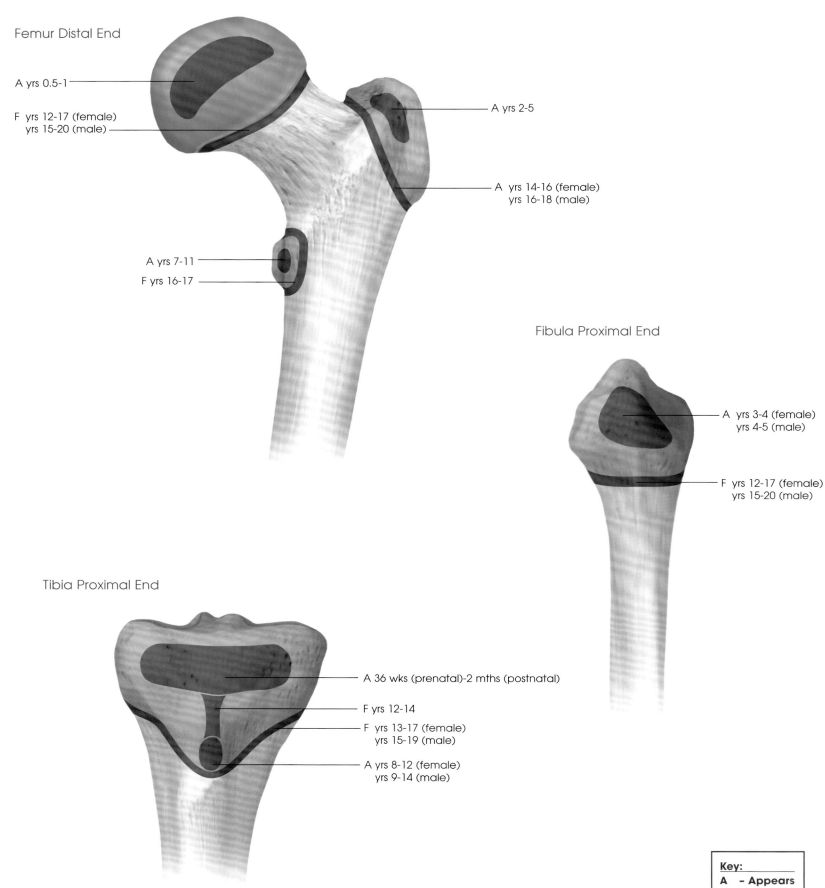

Femur Distal End

A yrs 0.5-1

F yrs 12-17 (female)
yrs 15-20 (male)

A yrs 2-5

A yrs 14-16 (female)
yrs 16-18 (male)

A yrs 7-11

F yrs 16-17

Fibula Proximal End

A yrs 3-4 (female)
yrs 4-5 (male)

F yrs 12-17 (female)
yrs 15-20 (male)

Tibia Proximal End

A 36 wks (prenatal)-2 mths (postnatal)

F yrs 12-14

F yrs 13-17 (female)
yrs 15-19 (male)

A yrs 8-12 (female)
yrs 9-14 (male)

Key:
A – Appears
F – Fuses

Extensor Mechanism Problems (children)

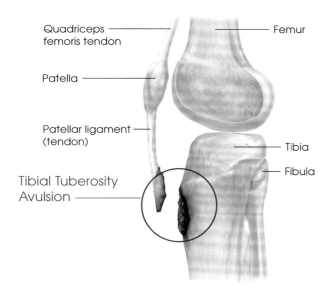

Quadriceps femoris tendon

Femur

Patella

Patellar ligament (tendon)

Tibial Tuberosity Avulsion

Tibia

Fibula

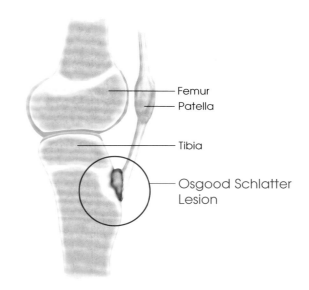

Femur

Patella

Tibia

Osgood Schlatter Lesion

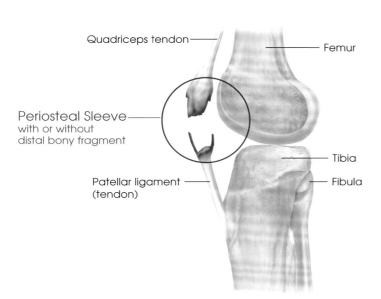

Quadriceps tendon

Femur

Periosteal Sleeve
with or without distal bony fragment

Tibia

Patellar ligament (tendon)

Fibula

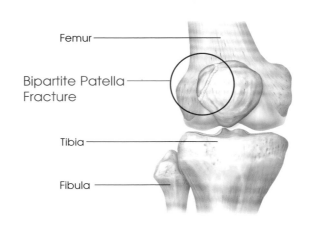

Femur

Bipartite Patella Fracture

Tibia

Fibula

Movements

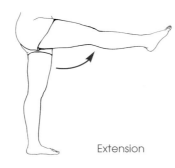

Extension

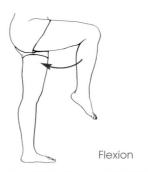

Flexion

Mechanism of Injury

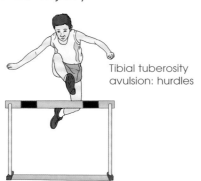

Tibial tuberosity avulsion: hurdles

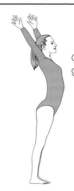

Osgood schlatter: gymnastics

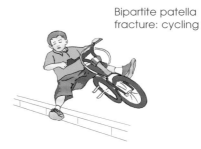

Bipartite patella fracture: cycling

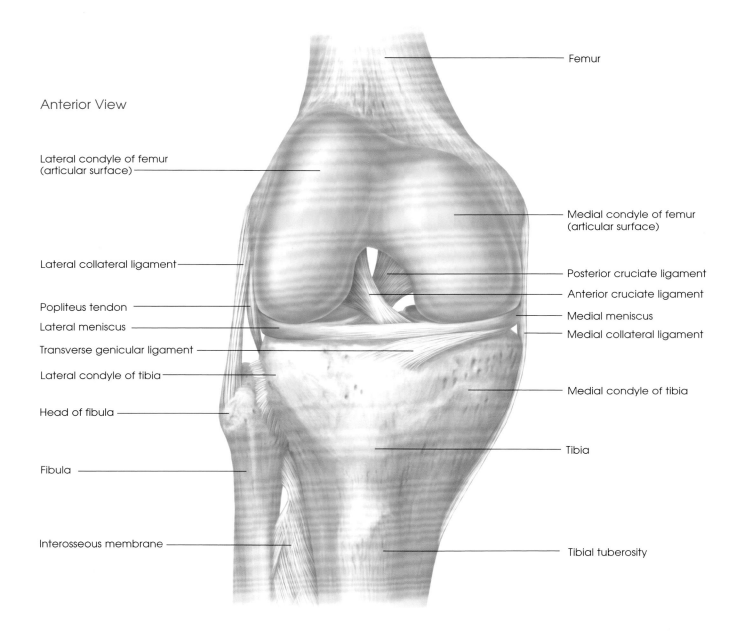

Anterior View

Femur

Lateral condyle of femur
(articular surface)

Medial condyle of femur
(articular surface)

Lateral collateral ligament

Posterior cruciate ligament

Anterior cruciate ligament

Popliteus tendon

Medial meniscus

Lateral meniscus

Medial collateral ligament

Transverse genicular ligament

Lateral condyle of tibia

Medial condyle of tibia

Head of fibula

Fibula

Tibia

Interosseous membrane

Tibial tuberosity

Fractures (adult) ——

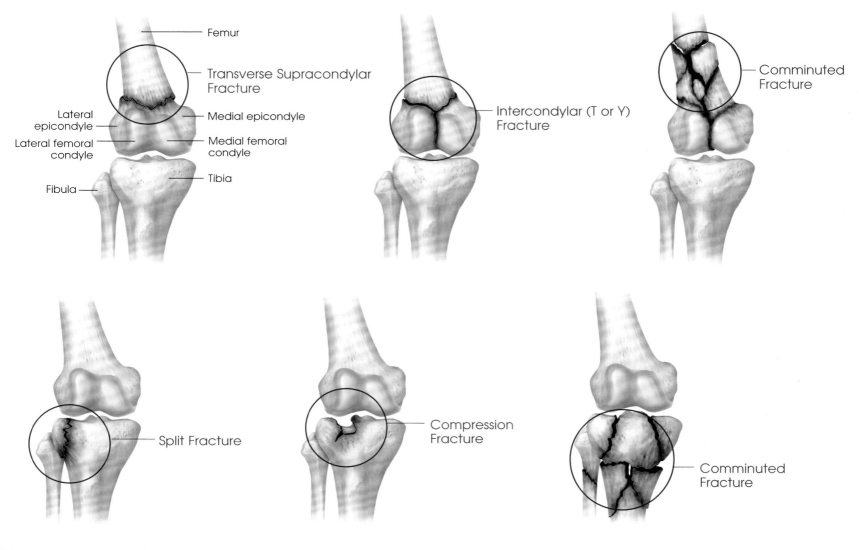

Femur

Transverse Supracondylar Fracture

Lateral epicondyle

Medial epicondyle

Lateral femoral condyle

Medial femoral condyle

Fibula

Tibia

Intercondylar (T or Y) Fracture

Comminuted Fracture

Split Fracture

Compression Fracture

Comminuted Fracture

Movements

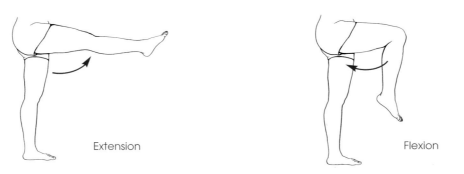

Extension

Flexion

Mechanism of Injury

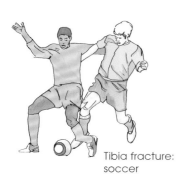

Tibia fracture: soccer

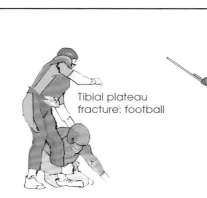

Tibial plateau fracture: football

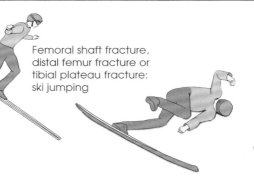

Femoral shaft fracture, distal femur fracture or tibial plateau fracture: ski jumping

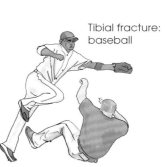

Tibial fracture: baseball

Proximal Femur

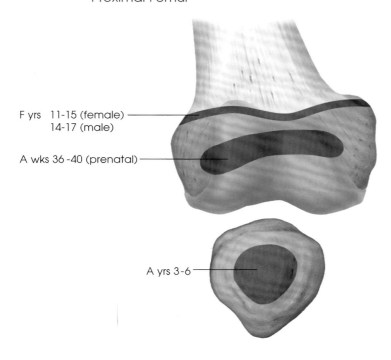

F yrs   11-15 (female)
           14-17 (male)

A wks 36 -40 (prenatal)

A yrs 3-6

Fibula Proximal End

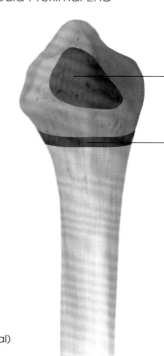

A yrs 3-4 (female)
    yrs 4-5 (male)

F yrs 12-17 (female)
    yrs 15-20 (male)

Tibia Proximal End

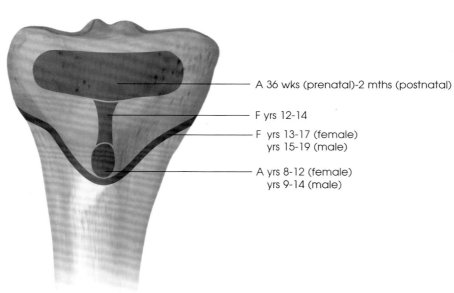

A 36 wks (prenatal)-2 mths (postnatal)

F yrs 12-14

F yrs 13-17 (female)
    yrs 15-19 (male)

A yrs 8-12 (female)
    yrs 9-14 (male)

Key:
A. **– Appears**
F.   **– Fuses**

Fractures (children)

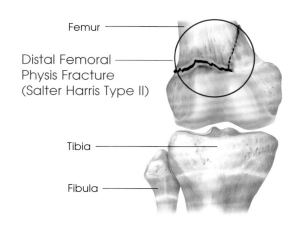

Femur

Distal Femoral
Physis Fracture
(Salter Harris Type II)

Tibia

Fibula

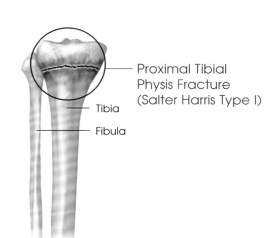

Proximal Tibial
Physis Fracture
(Salter Harris Type I)

Tibia

Fibula

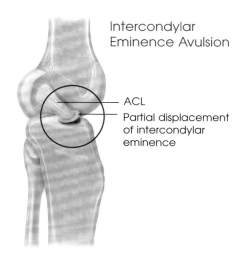

Intercondylar
Eminence Avulsion

ACL

Partial displacement
of intercondylar
eminence

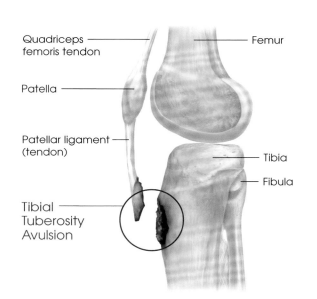

Quadriceps
femoris tendon

Patella

Patellar ligament
(tendon)

Femur

Tibia

Fibula

Tibial
Tuberosity
Avulsion

Salter-Harris Classification of Physis Injuries

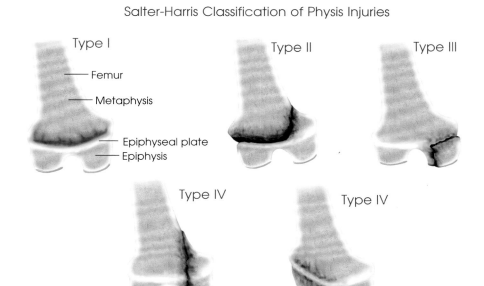

Type I

Femur

Metaphysis

Epiphyseal plate
Epiphysis

Type II

Type III

Type IV

Type IV

Movements

Extension

Flexion

Mechanism of Injury

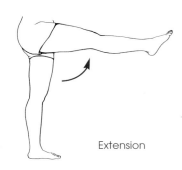

Distal femoral
physis fracture: football

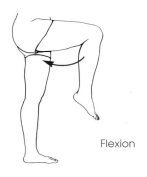

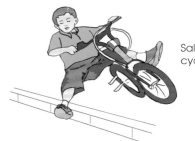

Salter Harris Fracture:
cycling

Right Knee, Anterior View

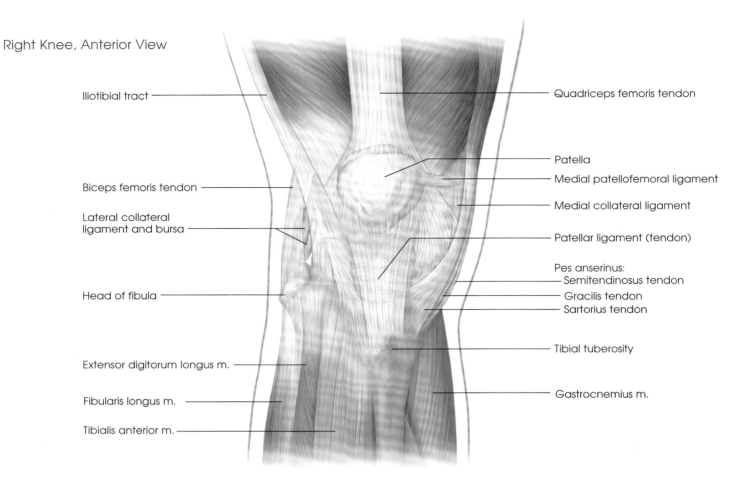

- Iliotibial tract
- Biceps femoris tendon
- Lateral collateral ligament and bursa
- Head of fibula
- Extensor digitorum longus m.
- Fibularis longus m.
- Tibialis anterior m.
- Quadriceps femoris tendon
- Patella
- Medial patellofemoral ligament
- Medial collateral ligament
- Patellar ligament (tendon)
- Pes anserinus:
  - Semitendinosus tendon
  - Gracilis tendon
  - Sartorius tendon
- Tibial tuberosity
- Gastrocnemius m.

Right Knee, Posterior View

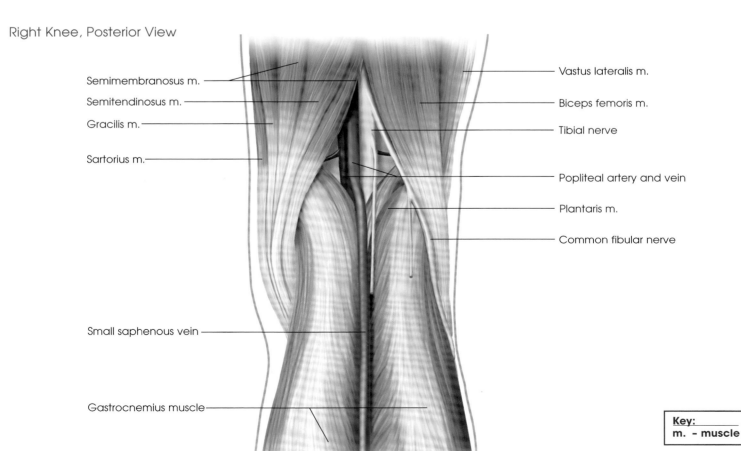

- Semimembranosus m.
- Semitendinosus m.
- Gracilis m.
- Sartorius m.
- Small saphenous vein
- Gastrocnemius muscle
- Vastus lateralis m.
- Biceps femoris m.
- Tibial nerve
- Popliteal artery and vein
- Plantaris m.
- Common fibular nerve

Key:
m. – muscle

Inflammations ⏤ | Knee |

Pathologies

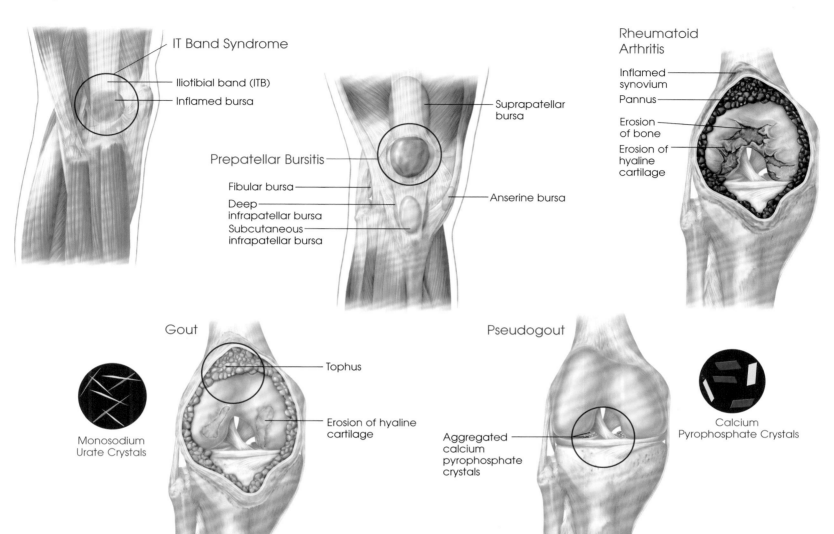

IT Band Syndrome
- Iliotibial band (ITB)
- Inflamed bursa

Prepatellar Bursitis
- Suprapatellar bursa
- Fibular bursa
- Deep infrapatellar bursa
- Subcutaneous infrapatellar bursa
- Anserine bursa

Rheumatoid Arthritis
- Inflamed synovium
- Pannus
- Erosion of bone
- Erosion of hyaline cartilage

Gout
- Tophus
- Erosion of hyaline cartilage

Monosodium Urate Crystals

Pseudogout
- Aggregated calcium pyrophosphate crystals

Calcium Pyrophosphate Crystals

Movements

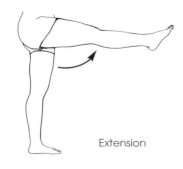

Extension

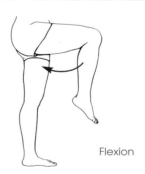

Flexion

Mechanism of Injury

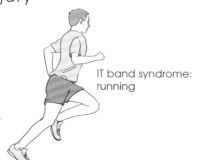

IT band syndrome: running

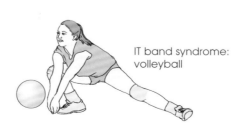

IT band syndrome: volleyball

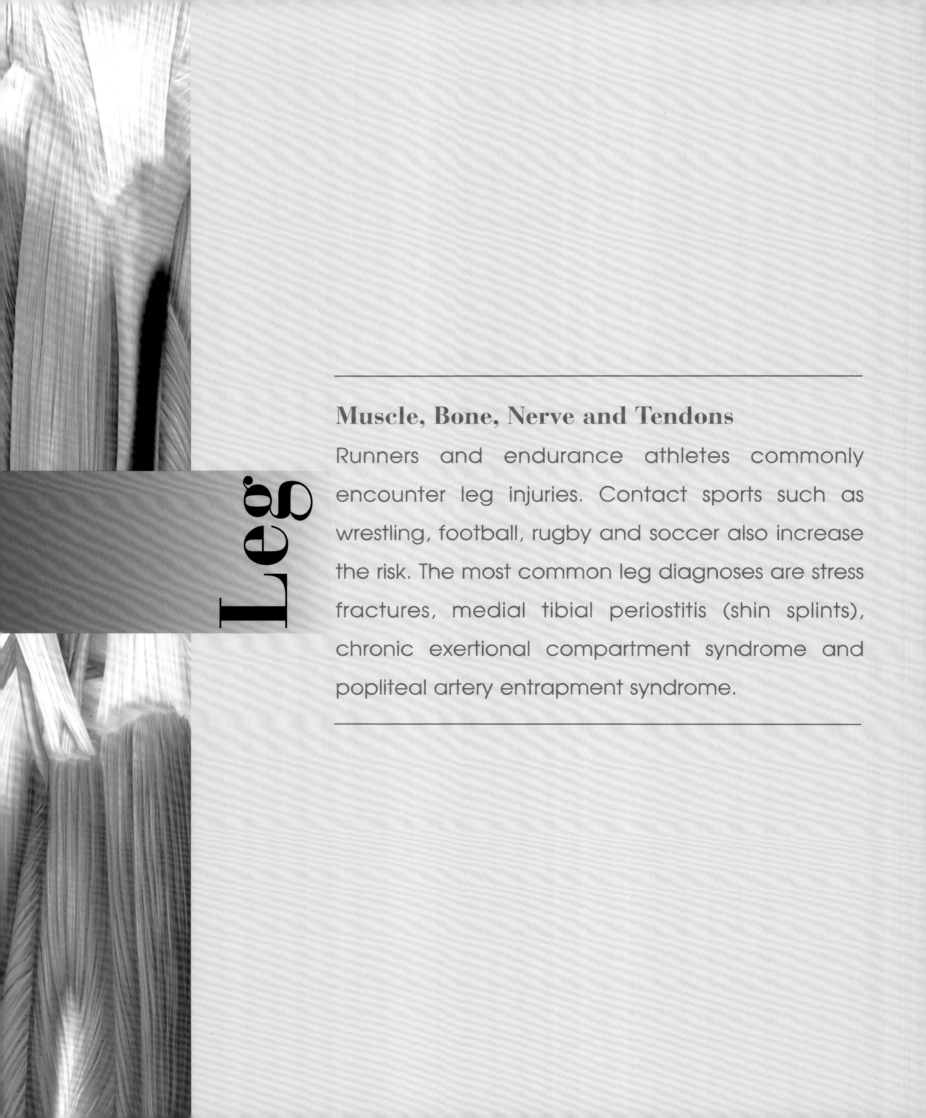

Leg

Muscle, Bone, Nerve and Tendons

Runners and endurance athletes commonly encounter leg injuries. Contact sports such as wrestling, football, rugby and soccer also increase the risk. The most common leg diagnoses are stress fractures, medial tibial periostitis (shin splints), chronic exertional compartment syndrome and popliteal artery entrapment syndrome.

chapter **8**

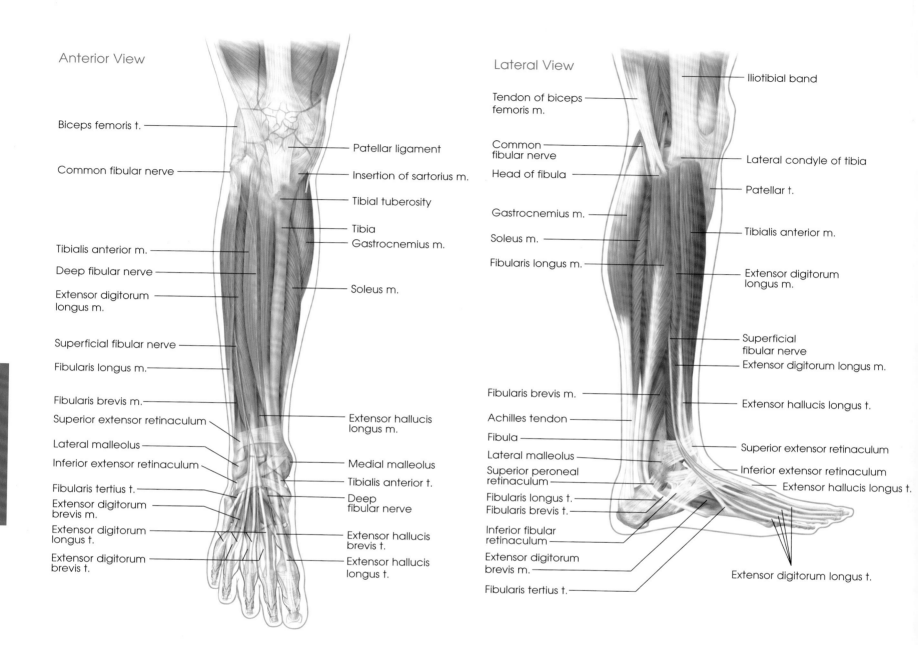

Anterior View

Biceps femoris t.

Common fibular nerve

Tibialis anterior m.

Deep fibular nerve

Extensor digitorum longus m.

Superficial fibular nerve

Fibularis longus m.

Fibularis brevis m.

Superior extensor retinaculum

Lateral malleolus

Inferior extensor retinaculum

Fibularis tertius t.

Extensor digitorum brevis m.

Extensor digitorum longus t.

Extensor digitorum brevis t.

Patellar ligament

Insertion of sartorius m.

Tibial tuberosity

Tibia

Gastrocnemius m.

Soleus m.

Extensor hallucis longus m.

Medial malleolus

Tibialis anterior t.

Deep fibular nerve

Extensor hallucis brevis t.

Extensor hallucis longus t.

Lateral View

Tendon of biceps femoris m.

Common fibular nerve

Head of fibula

Gastrocnemius m.

Soleus m.

Fibularis longus m.

Fibularis brevis m.

Achilles tendon

Fibula

Lateral malleolus

Superior peroneal retinaculum

Fibularis longus t.

Fibularis brevis t.

Inferior fibular retinaculum

Extensor digitorum brevis m.

Fibularis tertius t.

Iliotibial band

Lateral condyle of tibia

Patellar t.

Tibialis anterior m.

Extensor digitorum longus m.

Superficial fibular nerve

Extensor digitorum longus m.

Extensor hallucis longus t.

Superior extensor retinaculum

Inferior extensor retinaculum

Extensor hallucis longus t.

Extensor digitorum longus t.

Cross Section of the Right Leg

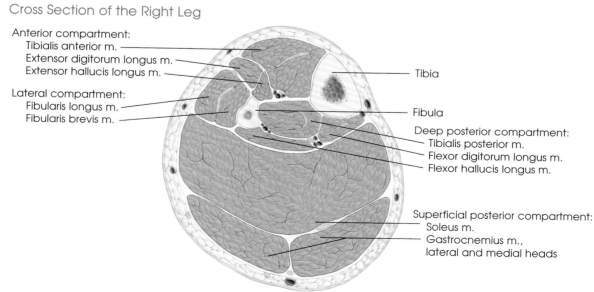

Anterior compartment:
Tibialis anterior m.
Extensor digitorum longus m.
Extensor hallucis longus m.

Lateral compartment:
Fibularis longus m.
Fibularis brevis m.

Tibia

Fibula

Deep posterior compartment:
Tibialis posterior m.
Flexor digitorum longus m.
Flexor hallucis longus m.

Superficial posterior compartment:
Soleus m.
Gastrocnemius m.,
lateral and medial heads

Key:
m. – muscle
t. – tendon

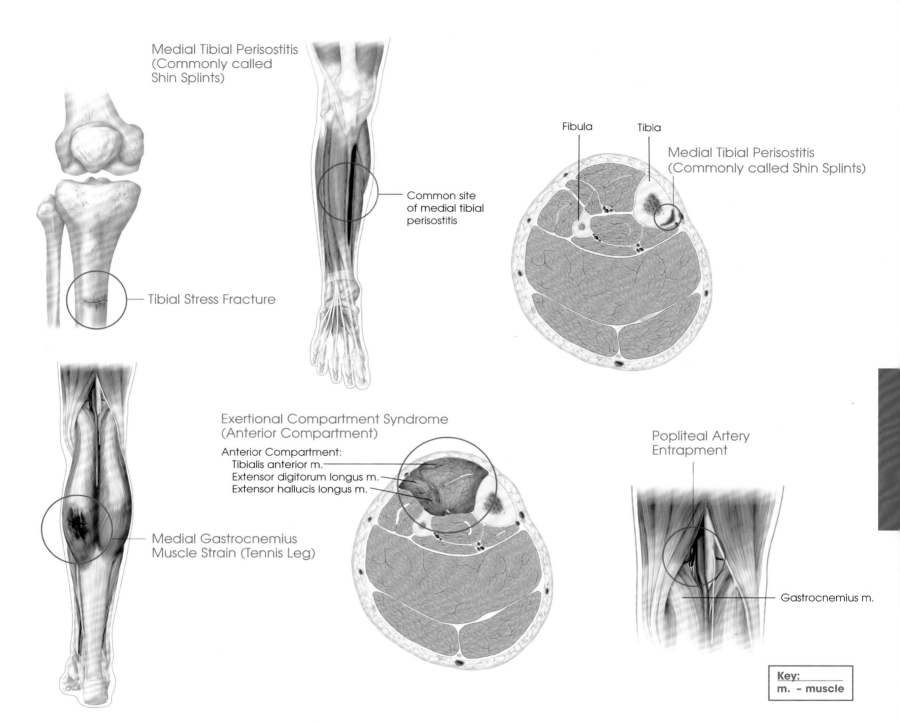

Medial Tibial Perisostitis (Commonly called Shin Splints)

Tibial Stress Fracture

Common site of medial tibial perisostitis

Fibula   Tibia

Medial Tibial Perisostitis (Commonly called Shin Splints)

Exertional Compartment Syndrome (Anterior Compartment)

Anterior Compartment:
Tibialis anterior m.
Extensor digitorum longus m.
Extensor hallucis longus m.

Medial Gastrocnemius Muscle Strain (Tennis Leg)

Popliteal Artery Entrapment

Gastrocnemius m.

Key:
m. – muscle

Mechanism of Injury

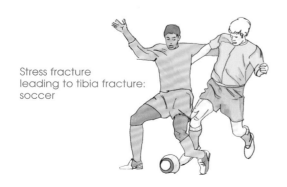

Stress fracture leading to tibia fracture: soccer

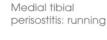

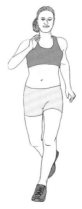

Medial tibial perisostitis: running

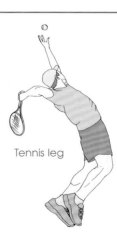

Tennis leg

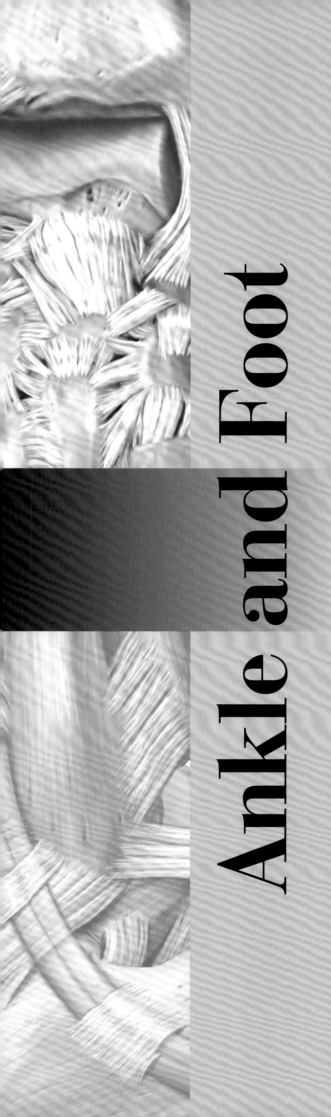

Ankle and Foot

The Base of Motor Activities

Strong enough to bear the body's weight, the foot and ankle form the base of all motor activities in sports; whether it be a sprinter pushing off from the blocks, a diver bouncing on a diving board or a gymnast landing a dismount. An accurate diagnosis of injury depends on a thorough understanding of the intricate foot and ankle anatomy.

chapter 9

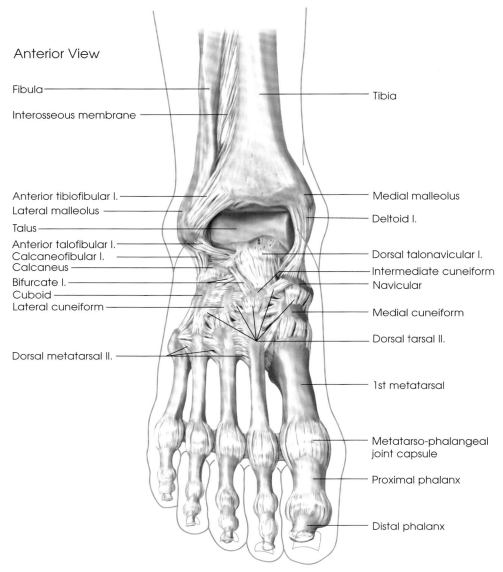

Anterior View

Fibula

Tibia

Interosseous membrane

Anterior tibiofibular l.

Medial malleolus

Lateral malleolus

Deltoid l.

Talus

Anterior talofibular l.

Dorsal talonavicular l.

Calcaneofibular l.

Intermediate cuneiform

Calcaneus

Navicular

Bifurcate l.

Cuboid

Medial cuneiform

Lateral cuneiform

Dorsal tarsal ll.

Dorsal metatarsal ll.

1st metatarsal

Metatarso-phalangeal joint capsule

Proximal phalanx

Distal phalanx

Lateral View

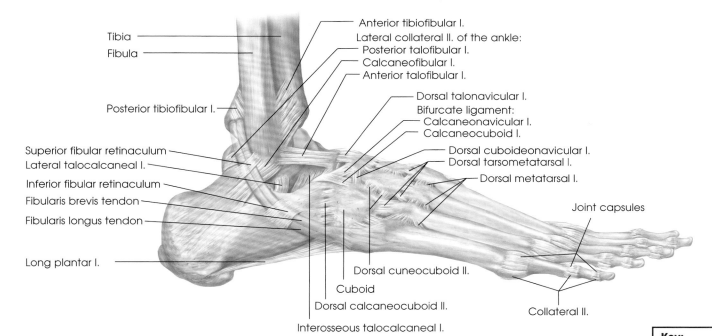

Tibia

Anterior tibiofibular l.

Lateral collateral ll. of the ankle:

Fibula

Posterior talofibular l.

Calcaneofibular l.

Anterior talofibular l.

Posterior tibiofibular l.

Dorsal talonavicular l.

Bifurcate ligament:

Calcaneonavicular l.

Calcaneocuboid l.

Superior fibular retinaculum

Dorsal cuboideonavicular l.

Lateral talocalcaneal l.

Dorsal tarsometatarsal l.

Inferior fibular retinaculum

Dorsal metatarsal l.

Fibularis brevis tendon

Joint capsules

Fibularis longus tendon

Long plantar l.

Dorsal cuneocuboid ll.

Cuboid

Collateral ll.

Dorsal calcaneocuboid ll.

Interosseous talocalcaneal l.

Key:
l. – ligament
ll. – ligaments

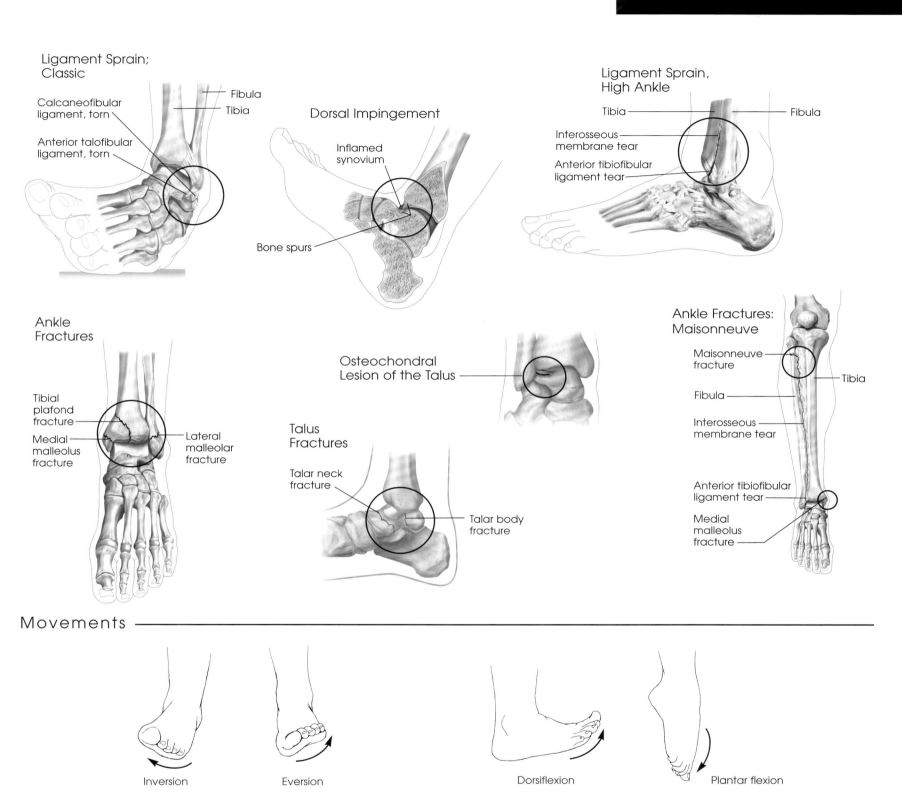

Ligament Sprain; Classic

- Fibula
- Tibia
- Calcaneofibular ligament, torn
- Anterior talofibular ligament, torn

Dorsal Impingement

- Inflamed synovium
- Bone spurs

Ligament Sprain, High Ankle

- Tibia
- Fibula
- Interosseous membrane tear
- Anterior tibiofibular ligament tear

Ankle Fractures

- Tibial plafond fracture
- Medial malleolus fracture
- Lateral malleolar fracture

Osteochondral Lesion of the Talus

Talus Fractures

- Talar neck fracture
- Talar body fracture

Ankle Fractures: Maisonneuve

- Maisonneuve fracture
- Tibia
- Fibula
- Interosseous membrane tear
- Anterior tibiofibular ligament tear
- Medial malleolus fracture

Movements

- Inversion
- Eversion
- Dorsiflexion
- Plantar flexion

Mechanism of Injury

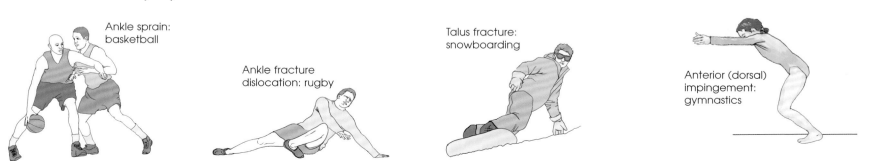

- Ankle sprain: basketball
- Ankle fracture dislocation: rugby
- Talus fracture: snowboarding
- Anterior (dorsal) impingement: gymnastics

—Normal Anatomy–
Growth Plates and Ossification Sites

Distal Tibia and Fibula,
Anterior View

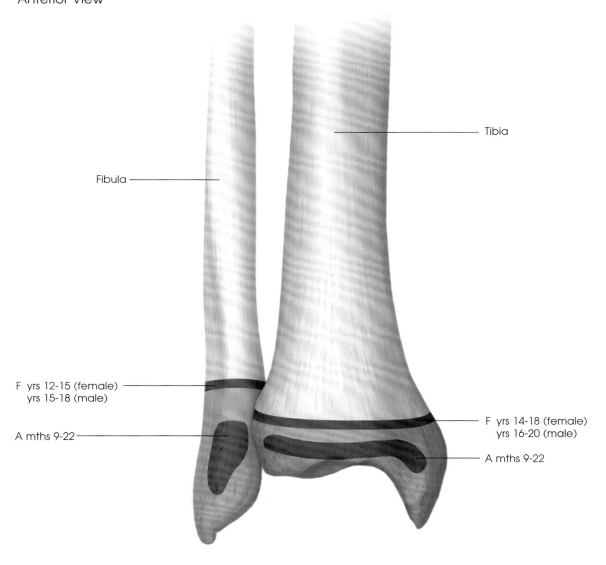

Tibia

Fibula

F yrs 12-15 (female)
yrs 15-18 (male)

A mths 9-22

F yrs 14-18 (female)
yrs 16-20 (male)

A mths 9-22

Key:
A   – Appears
F   – Fuses

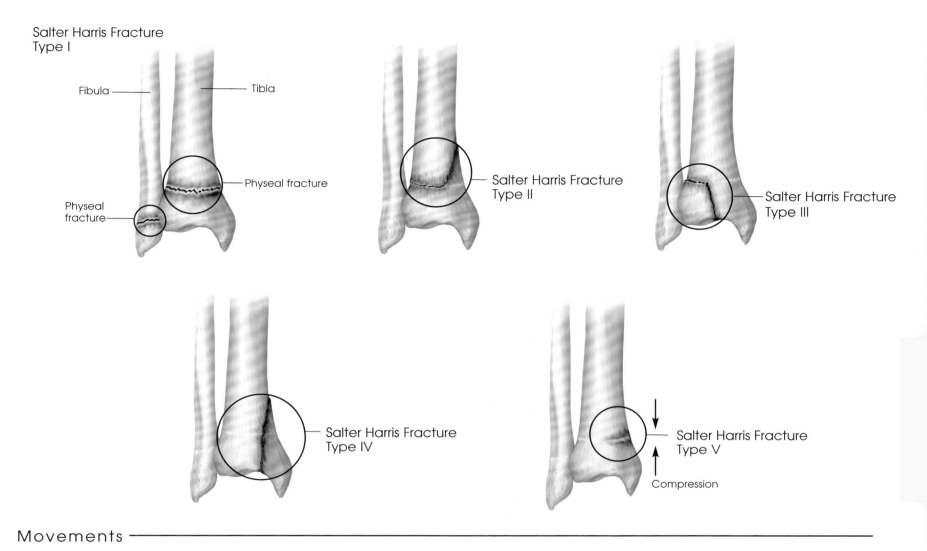

Salter Harris Fracture
Type I

Fibula — — Tibia

— Physeal fracture

Physeal
fracture —

Salter Harris Fracture
Type II

Salter Harris Fracture
Type III

Salter Harris Fracture
Type IV

Salter Harris Fracture
Type V

Compression

Movements

Inversion

Eversion

Dorsiflexion

Plantar flexion

Mechanism of Injury

While the mechanism is the same, physeal and not ligament or main bone body fractures are more common in children.

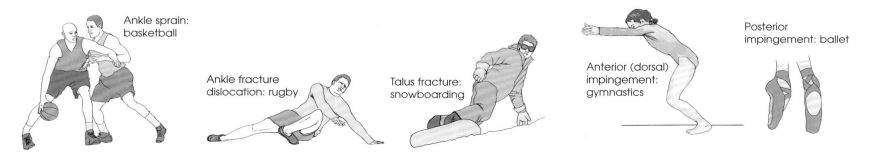

Ankle sprain:
basketball

Ankle fracture
dislocation: rugby

Talus fracture:
snowboarding

Anterior (dorsal)
impingement:
gymnastics

Posterior
impingement: ballet

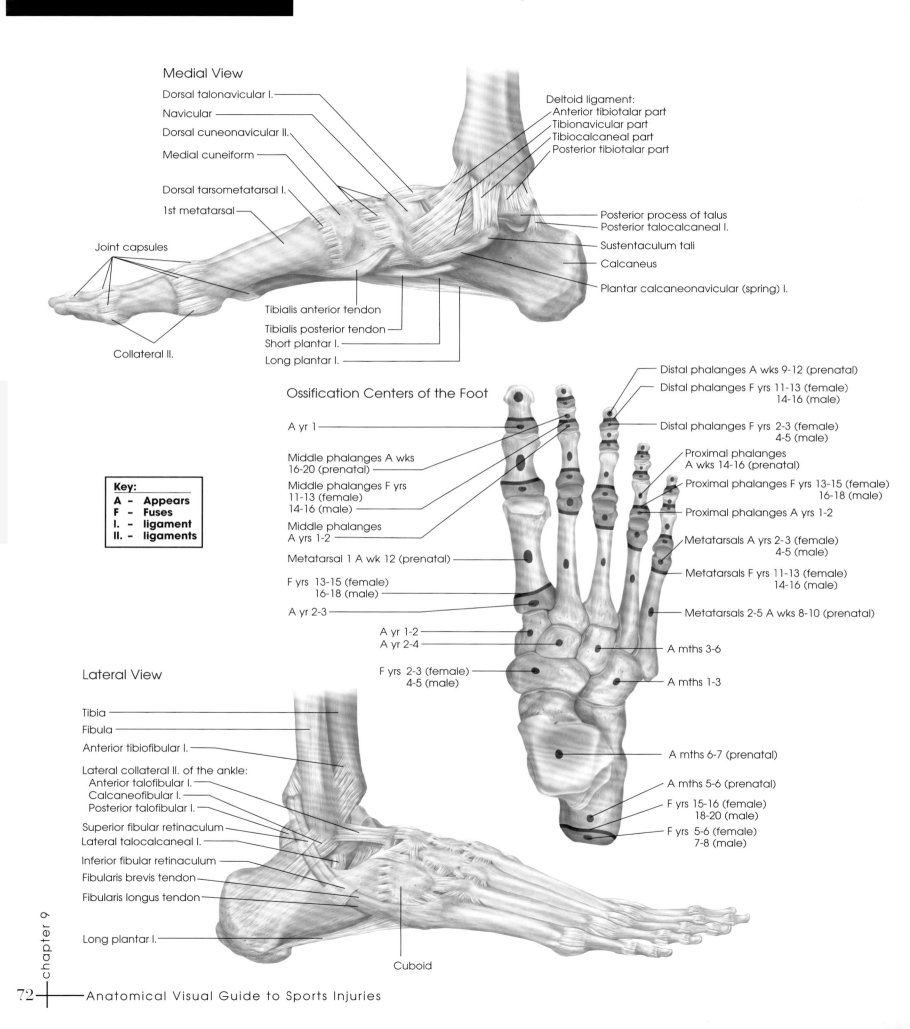

Medial View

Dorsal talonavicular l.
Navicular
Dorsal cuneonavicular ll.
Medial cuneiform
Dorsal tarsometatarsal l.
1st metatarsal
Joint capsules
Collateral ll.

Deltoid ligament:
Anterior tibiotalar part
Tibionavicular part
Tibiocalcaneal part
Posterior tibiotalar part

Posterior process of talus
Posterior talocalcaneal l.
Sustentaculum tali
Calcaneus
Plantar calcaneonavicular (spring) l.

Tibialis anterior tendon
Tibialis posterior tendon
Short plantar l.
Long plantar l.

Ossification Centers of the Foot

Distal phalanges A wks 9-12 (prenatal)
Distal phalanges F yrs 11-13 (female)
14-16 (male)
Distal phalanges F yrs 2-3 (female)
4-5 (male)

A yr 1

Middle phalanges A wks
16-20 (prenatal)
Middle phalanges F yrs
11-13 (female)
14-16 (male)
Middle phalanges
A yrs 1-2

Proximal phalanges
A wks 14-16 (prenatal)
Proximal phalanges F yrs 13-15 (female)
16-18 (male)
Proximal phalanges A yrs 1-2

Metatarsals A yrs 2-3 (female)
4-5 (male)

Metatarsal 1 A wk 12 (prenatal)

F yrs 13-15 (female)
16-18 (male)

A yr 2-3

Metatarsals F yrs 11-13 (female)
14-16 (male)

Metatarsals 2-5 A wks 8-10 (prenatal)

A yr 1-2
A yr 2-4
F yrs 2-3 (female)
4-5 (male)

A mths 3-6
A mths 1-3

Key:
A – **Appears**
F – **Fuses**
l. – **ligament**
ll. – **ligaments**

Lateral View

Tibia
Fibula
Anterior tibiofibular l.
Lateral collateral ll. of the ankle:
Anterior talofibular l.
Calcaneofibular l.
Posterior talofibular l.
Superior fibular retinaculum
Lateral talocalcaneal l.
Inferior fibular retinaculum
Fibularis brevis tendon
Fibularis longus tendon

Long plantar l.

A mths 6-7 (prenatal)

A mths 5-6 (prenatal)

F yrs 15-16 (female)
18-20 (male)

F yrs 5-6 (female)
7-8 (male)

Cuboid

Hindfoot Injuries
(children & adult)

Tarsal Tunnel,
Calcaneal Fracture,
Plantar Fasciitis

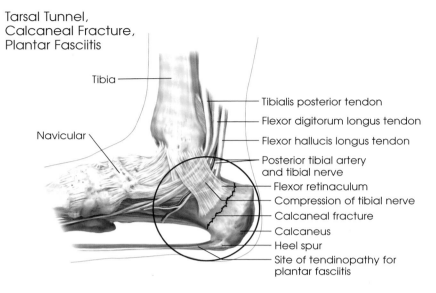

Tibia

Tibialis posterior tendon

Flexor digitorum longus tendon

Navicular

Flexor hallucis longus tendon

Posterior tibial artery and tibial nerve

Flexor retinaculum

Compression of tibial nerve

Calcaneal fracture

Calcaneus

Heel spur

Site of tendinopathy for plantar fasciitis

Achilles Tendon Rupture

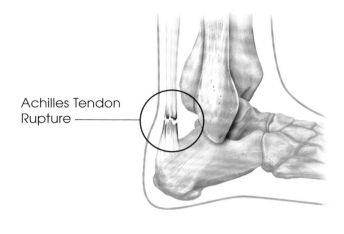

Tibia

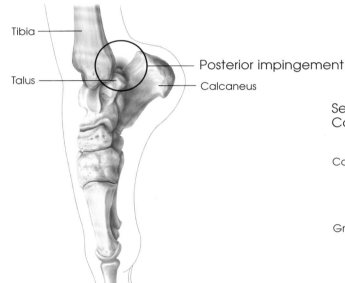

Talus

Posterior impingement

Calcaneus

Sever's Disease:
Calcaneal Apophysitis in Children

Calcaneus

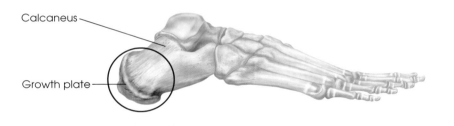

Growth plate

Movements

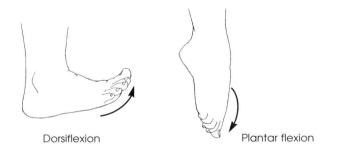

Inversion   Eversion   Dorsiflexion   Plantar flexion

Mechanism of Injury

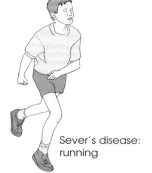

Sever's disease:
running

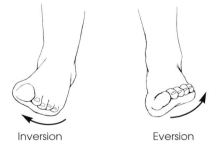

Anterior (dorsal) impingement: gymnastics

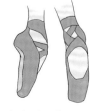

Posterior impingement: ballet

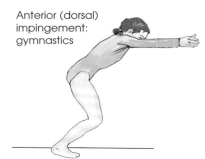

Tarsal tunnel: running

 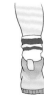

Achilles tendonitis: basketball

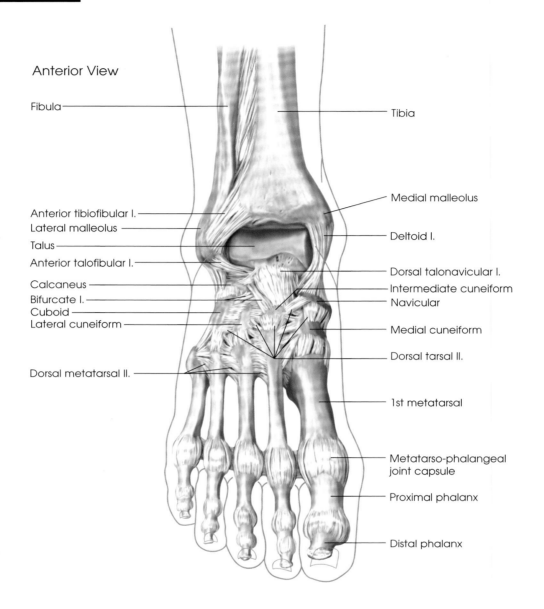

Anterior View

Fibula

Tibia

Anterior tibiofibular I.

Medial malleolus

Lateral malleolus

Deltoid I.

Talus

Anterior talofibular I.

Dorsal talonavicular I.

Calcaneus

Intermediate cuneiform

Bifurcate I.

Navicular

Cuboid

Lateral cuneiform

Medial cuneiform

Dorsal tarsal II.

Dorsal metatarsal II.

1st metatarsal

Metatarso-phalangeal joint capsule

Proximal phalanx

Distal phalanx

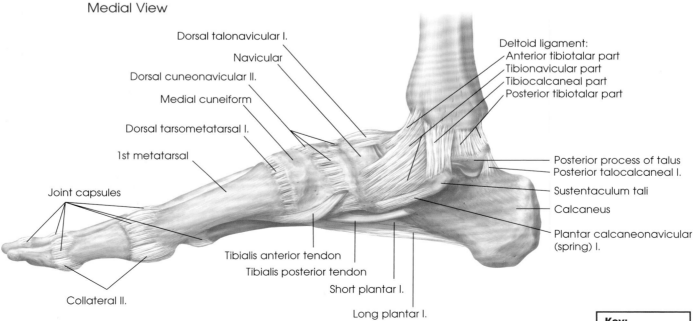

Medial View

Dorsal talonavicular I.

Navicular

Dorsal cuneonavicular II.

Medial cuneiform

Dorsal tarsometatarsal I.

1st metatarsal

Joint capsules

Deltoid ligament:
Anterior tibiotalar part
Tibionavicular part
Tibiocalcaneal part
Posterior tibiotalar part

Posterior process of talus
Posterior talocalcaneal I.

Sustentaculum tali

Calcaneus

Plantar calcaneonavicular (spring) I.

Tibialis anterior tendon

Tibialis posterior tendon

Short plantar I.

Collateral II.

Long plantar I.

Key:
I. – ligament
II. – ligaments

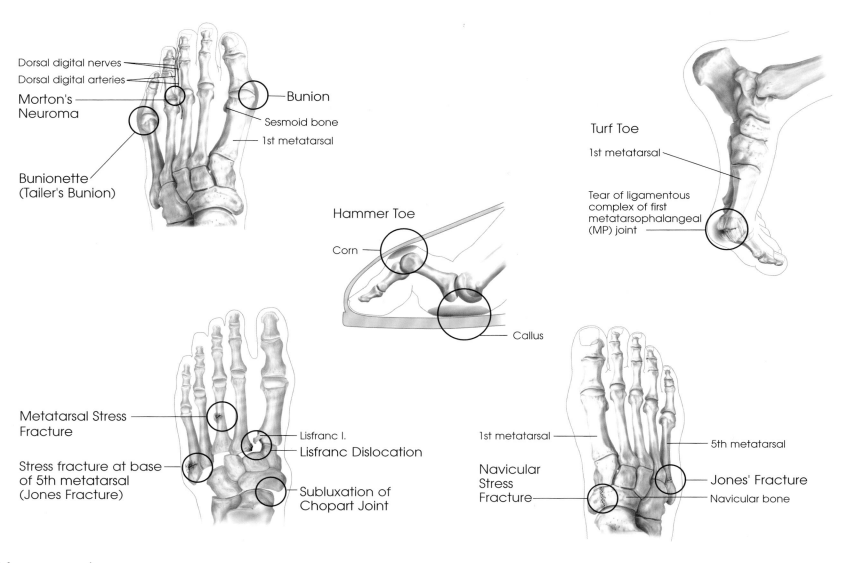

Dorsal digital nerves
Dorsal digital arteries
Morton's Neuroma
Bunionette (Tailer's Bunion)

Bunion
Sesmoid bone
1st metatarsal

Hammer Toe
Corn
Callus

Turf Toe
1st metatarsal
Tear of ligamentous complex of first metatarsophalangeal (MP) joint

Metatarsal Stress Fracture
Stress fracture at base of 5th metatarsal (Jones Fracture)
Lisfranc I.
Lisfranc Dislocation
Subluxation of Chopart Joint

1st metatarsal
Navicular Stress Fracture
5th metatarsal
Jones' Fracture
Navicular bone

Movements ─────────────────

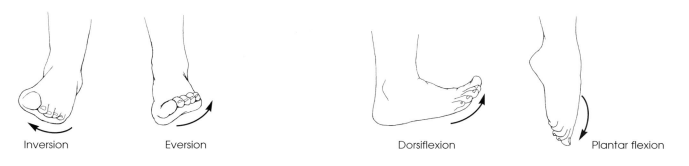

Inversion Eversion Dorsiflexion Plantar flexion

Mechanism of Injury ─────────────

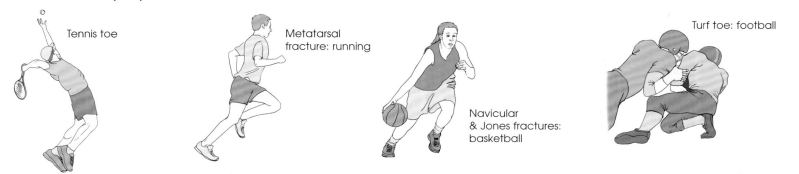

Tennis toe
Metatarsal fracture: running
Navicular & Jones fractures: basketball
Turf toe: football

Coronal sutu
Frontal

Nasal
Lacrima
Ethm
Sphe
Zyg
Infra
Maxilla
Lateral
Articul
Mandib
Mental

us
chae
s (C1)
is (C2)

Hyoid

Styloid process
Stylomandibula
*Gravity line emer,
from body of C7*

Clavicle
1st rib
Manu

Anatomical Charts

The Sum of the Parts

A study of one part of the body cannot be done without a knowledge of the workings of the whole. These anatomical charts offer a detailed look at the body's various systems, and at the same time, provide a broader view of the body's framework, its mechanisms and its ability to function as a whole.

Anterior View

Skin
alis m.

ularis
li m.:
part
art

n.
m.

ticus
ajor m.
sseter m.
inator m.
Depressor
ali oris m.
sor labii
ris m.

Galea aponeuroti
Frontalis m.
Corrugate
supercili
Levator
superio
alaeque
Auricula
Supe
Ant
Leva
labii
superi
Zygom
minor m
Risorius m
Levator an,
oris m.
Depressor s
Orbicularis
Mentalis
Om

3
3

9
10
9

chapter **10**

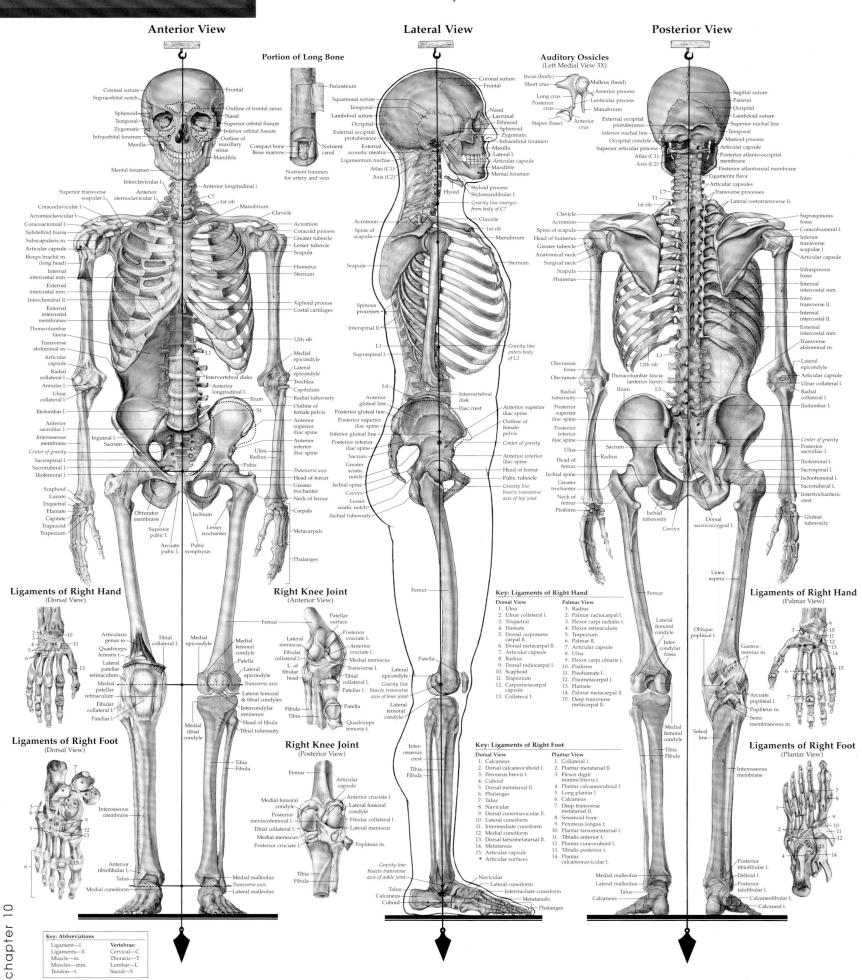

The Muscular System

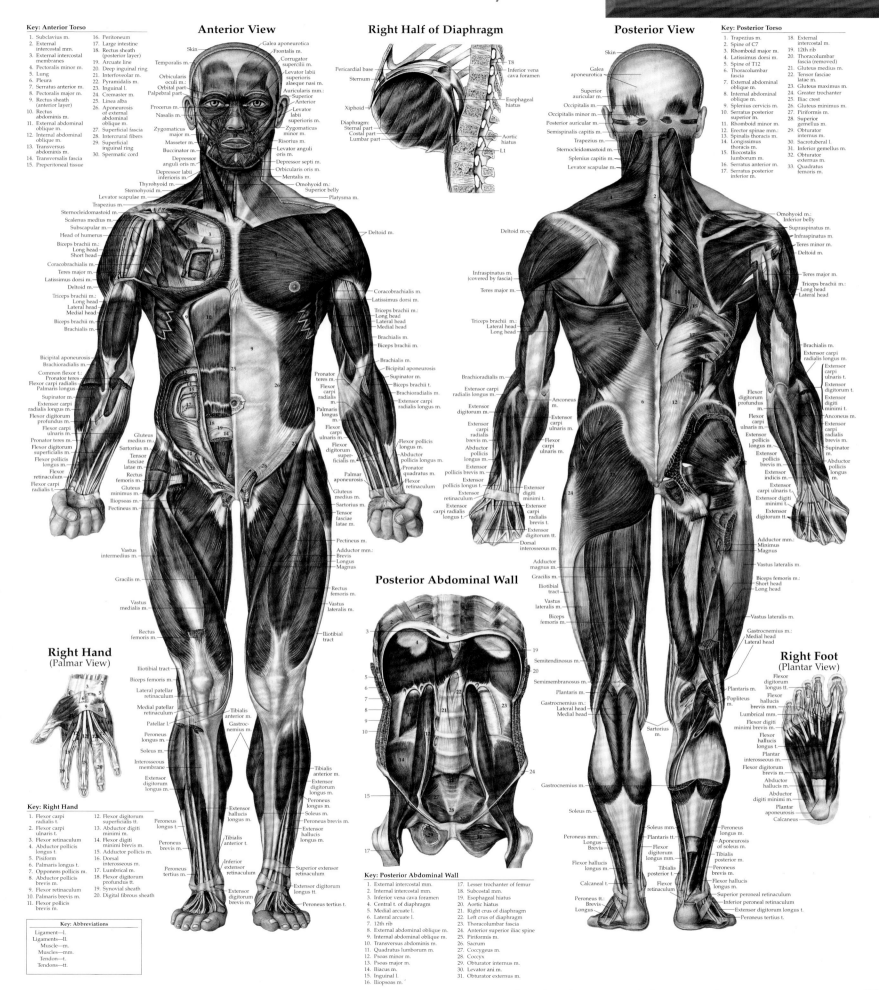

Anterior View

Right Half of Diaphragm

Posterior View

Posterior Abdominal Wall

Right Hand (Palmar View)

Right Foot (Plantar View)

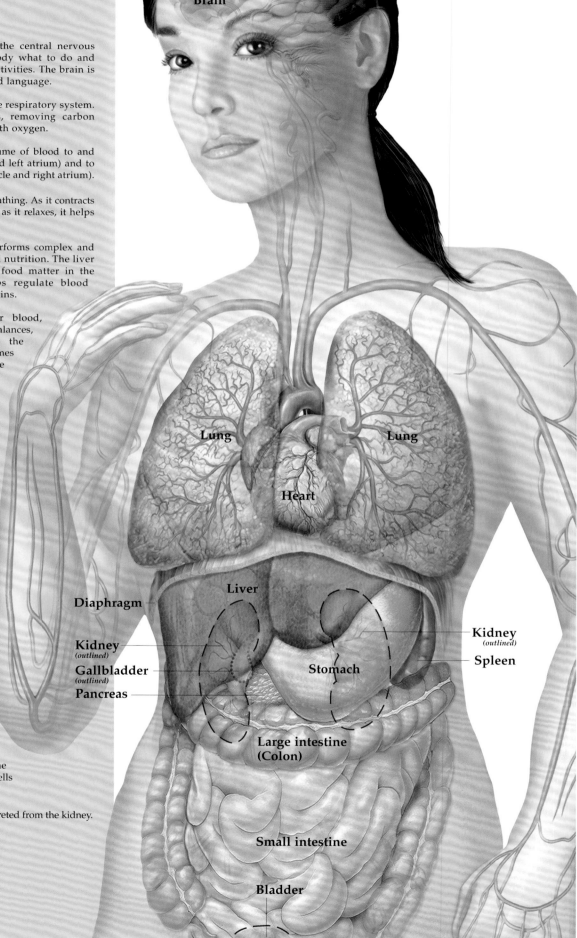

The brain is the command center of the central nervous system. It receives signals that tell the body what to do and controls both voluntary and involuntary activities. The brain is the home of emotion, memory, thought, and language.

The lungs are the main component of the respiratory system. They distribute air and exchange gases, removing carbon dioxide from the blood and providing it with oxygen.

The heart pumps the body's entire volume of blood to and from the lungs (using the right ventricle and left atrium) and to and from all the organs (using the left ventricle and right atrium).

The diaphragm plays a vital role in breathing. As it contracts and flattens, it helps draw air into the lungs; as it relaxes, it helps push the air out of the lungs.

The liver, the largest internal organ performs complex and important functions related to digestion and nutrition. The liver produces bile (which helps break down food matter in the small intestine), detoxifies blood, helps regulate blood glucose levels, and produces plasma proteins.

The kidneys eliminate waste, filter blood, maintain fluid-electrolyte and acid-base balances, produce the hormone that stimulates the production of red blood cells, produce enzymes that govern blood pressure, and help activate vitamin D.

The spleen breaks down old red blood cells and selectively retains and destroys damaged or abnormal red blood cells. It also filters out bacteria and other foreign substances that enter the bloodstream. The spleen stores blood and produces cells involved in immune response.

The gallbladder stores the bile that is secreted by the liver.

The pancreas assists with the digestion of many substances such as protein, nucleic acids, starch, fats and cholesterol. Using the hormone insulin, the pancreas controls the amount of sugar stored in and released from the liver for use throughout the body.

The stomach temporarily stores food and begins the digestion process, breaking down the food with gastric acids and moving it into the small intestine.

The large intestine absorbs water, secretes mucus, and eliminates digestive waste.

The small intestine completes digestion. Food molecules are absorbed through the wall of the intestine into the circulatory system and delivered to the cells of the body.

The bladder stores urine that has been excreted from the kidney.

Heart (Right interior view)

Right brachiocephalic v.
Left brachiocephalic v.
Superior vena cava
Left subclavian a.
Left common carotid a.
Brachiocephalic trunk
Arch of aorta
Ligamentum arteriosum
Pulmonary trunk
Pulmonary valve:
Right semilunar cusp
Anterior semilunar cusp
Left semilunar cusp
Reflection of pericardium
Right auricle
Pectinate muscles
Fossa ovalis
Conus arteriosus
Left auricle
Supraventricular crest
Great cardiac v.
Anterior interventricular br. of the left coronary a.
Left ventricle
Chordae tendineae
Moderator band
Muscular interventricular septum
Crista terminalis
Right atrium
Right coronary a.
Tricuspid valve:
Anterior cusp
Septal cusp
Posterior cusp
Anterior papillary muscle
Hepatic vv.
Pericardial sac
Inferior vena cava
Abdominal aorta
Apex of heart
Limbus

Heart (Left interior view)

Aorta
Ligamentum arteriosum
Left coronary a.
Left superior pulmonary v.
Left auricle
Great cardiac v.
Circumflex br. of left coronary a.
Mitral valve:
Posterior cusp
Anterior cusp
Anterior papillary muscle
Interventricular septum
Trabeculae carneae
Azygos v.
Superior vena cava
Right pulmonary a.
Right superior pulmonary v.
Right inferior pulmonary v.
Interatrial septum
Valve of foramen ovale
Left inferior pulmonary v.
Chordae tendineae
Epicardium
Myocardium
Endocardium
Posterior papillary muscle

Heart (Posterior view)

Aorta
Ligamentum arteriosum
Left pulmonary a.
Left pulmonary vv.
Right pulmonary vv.
Left atrium
Left auricle
Oblique v. of left atrium
Great cardiac v.
Coronary sinus
Posterior vv. of left ventricle
Left subclavian a.
Left common carotid a.
Brachiocephalic trunk
Azygos v.
Superior vena cava
Right pulmonary a.
Right atrium
Pericardium
Interatrial sulcus
Inferior vena cava
Terminal sulcus
Small cardiac v.
Middle cardiac v.
Right atrium
Right coronary a.
Posterior interventricular sulcus
Left ventricle
Right ventricle
Apex of heart

Heart in Systole
(Superior view, atria removed)

Pulmonary trunk
Pulmonary valve:
Right semilunar cusp
Anterior semilunar cusp
Left semilunar cusp
Anterior interventricular a.
Circumflex br. of left coronary a.
Aortic valve:
Left semilunar cusp
Right semilunar cusp
Posterior semilunar cusp
Mitral valve:
Anterior cusp
Posterior cusp
Coronary sinus
Conus arteriosus
Right coronary a.
Tricuspid valve:
Anterior cusp
Septal cusp
Posterior cusp
Interatrial septum
Opening of middle cardiac v.

Female Pelvis
(Posterior view)

Uterine (fallopian) tube
Ovarian a.
Left common iliac a.
Femoral n.
Iliacus muscle
Left external iliac a.
Superior vesical a.
Superior gluteal a.
Inferior gluteal a.
Obturator a.
Uterine a.
Inferior vesical a.
Vaginal a.
Left ureter
Internal pudendal a.
Inferior rectal a.
Urinary bladder
Sciatic n.
Ovaries
Uterine a.:
Tubal br.
Ovarian br.
Uterus
Superior gluteal a. & v.
Uterine a. & v.
Uterosacral ligament
Inferior gluteal a. & v.
Internal pudendal a. & vv.
Deep femoral a.
Medial circumflex femoral a.
Obturator internus muscle
Femoral a.
Right common iliac a.
Ovarian a. & vv.
Right external iliac a.
Right ureter
Levator ani muscle
Uterine a. (Vaginal brs.) Vagina
Uterovaginal venous plexus
1st perforating a.

Superficial temporal a. & v.
Frontal br.
Parietal br.
Middle temporal a. & v.
Middle meningeal a.
Superficial temporal a.
Maxillary a. & v.
Posterior auricular a.
Occipital a. & v.
Inferior alveolar a.
Posterior auricular v.
Retromandibular v.
External jugular v.
Internal jugular v.
Internal carotid a.
Vertebral a.
Transverse cervical a.
Inferior thyroid a.
Thyrocervical trunk
Costocervical trunk
Dorsal scapular a.
Suprascapular a.
Axillary a. & v.
Thoracoacromial a.
Subscapular a.
Anterior circumflex humeral a.
Posterior circumflex humeral a.
Scapular circumflex a.
Lateral thoracic a.
Thoracodorsal a.
Brachial a.
Deep brachial a.
Middle collateral a.
Radial collateral a.
Superior ulnar collateral a.
Inferior ulnar collateral a.
Interosseous recurrent a.
Radial recurrent a.
Anterior ulnar recurrent a.
Posterior ulnar recurrent a.
Common interosseous a.
Posterior interosseous a.
Anterior interosseous a.
Ulnar a.
Median a.
Interosseous membrane
Radial a.
Deep palmar br. of ulnar a.
Superficial palmar br. of radial a.
Deep palmar arch
Superficial palmar arch
Palmar metacarpal aa.
Common palmar digital aa.
Proper palmar digital aa.

Supraorbital a.
Supratrochlear a.
Dorsal nasal a.
Deep temporal aa.
Infraorbital a.
Angular v.
Posterior superior alveolar a.
Buccal a.
Masseteric a.
Superior labial a. & v.
Inferior labial a. & v.
Facial a. & v.
Submental a. & v.
Lingual a. & v.
Superior laryngeal a. & v.
Superior thyroid aa. & vv.
Internal jugular v.
External jugular v.
Middle thyroid v.
Transverse cervical v.
1st rib
Suprascapular v.
Dorsal scapular v.
Subclavian a. & v.
Cephalic v.
Lateral thoracic a. & vv.
Anterior circumflex humeral a. & vv.
Posterior circumflex humeral a. & vv.
Scapular circumflex a. & v.
Brachial a. & v.
Thoracodorsal a. & v.
Basilic v.
Deep brachial a. & v.
Radial collateral a. & v.
Superior ulnar collateral a. & vv.
Middle collateral a. & vv.
Basilic v.
Cephalic v.
Brachial a. & vv.
Radial recurrent a.
Median cubital v.
Accessory cephalic v.
Radial a. & vv.
Ulnar a. & vv.
Anterior interosseous a. & v.
Median antebrachial v.
Ulnar a. & v.:
Deep palmar br.
Deep palmar arch
Superficial palmar arch
Radial a. & vv.:
Superficial palmar br.
Intercapitular vv.
Proper palmar digital vv.

Inferior gluteal a.
Medial circumflex femoral a.
Lateral circumflex femoral a.:
Ascending br.
Descending br.
Sciatic n.
Deep femoral a.
1st perforating a. & v.
2nd perforating a.
3rd perforating a.
4th perforating a.
Popliteal a.
Lateral superior genicular a.
Sural aa.
Middle genicular a.
Lateral inferior genicular a.
Anterior recurrent tibial a. & vv.
Anterior tibial a.
Posterior tibial a. & vv.
Peroneal a.
Interosseous membrane
Anterior medial malleolar a.
Anterior lateral malleolar a.
Lateral tarsal a.
Medial tarsal a.
Lateral plantar a.
Medial plantar a.
Arcuate a.
Deep plantar a.
Dorsal digital aa.

Femoral a. & v.
Descending br. of lateral circumflex femoral a. & v.
2nd perforating a. & v.
3rd perforating a. & v.
Adductor hiatus
Descending genicular a.:
Articular br.
Saphenous br.
Medial superior genicular a. & v.
Medial inferior genicular a. & vv.
Lesser saphenous v.
Lateral superior genicular a. & vv.
Sural aa. & vv.
Lateral inferior genicular a. & vv.
Popliteal a.
Great saphenous v.
Perforating br. of peroneal a.
Great saphenous v.
Dorsalis pedis a. & vv.
Dorsal venous rete
Dorsal venous arch
Dorsal metatarsal vv.
Dorsal digital vv.
Dorsal metatarsal aa.

Base of the Brain
(Left cerebellum removed)

Branches of anterior cerebral aa.
Optic n. (II)
Anterior cerebral a.
Lateral sulcus
Internal carotid a.
Middle cerebral a.
Lenticulostriate aa.
Pituitary gland
Posterior communicating a.
Oculomotor n. (III)
Superior cerebellar a.
Basilar a.
Medulla oblongata
Ventral root of C1
Spinal cord
Olfactory tract (I)
Anterior communicating a.
Optic tract
Anterior choroidal a.
Mamillary body
Posterior cerebral a.
Pons
Anterior inferior cerebellar a.
Vagus n. (X)
Anterior spinal a.
Posterior inferior cerebellar a.
Vertebral a.
Cerebellum
Accessory n. (XI)

Key: Central Figure

1. Parietal pleura
2. Right internal thoracic a. & v.
3. Right brachiocephalic v.
4. Brachiocephalic trunk
5. Left common carotid a.
6. Superior vena cava
7. Pericardium
8. Ascending aorta
9. Pulmonary trunk
10. Left pulmonary a.
11. Right lung
12. Right atrium and auricle
13. Left auricle
14. Left pulmonary a.
15. Right coronary a.
16. Anterior interventricular a.
17. Diaphragm
18. Hepatic vv.
19. Inferior vena cava
20. Inferior phrenic aa.
21. Superior suprarenal aa.
22. Right suprarenal gland
23. Middle and inferior suprarenal aa.
24. Right kidney
25. Testicular aa. & vv.
26. 10th rib
27. Abdominal aorta
28. Inferior mesenteric a.
29. Ascending lumbar v.
30. Common iliac aa. & vv.
31. Anterior superior iliac spine
32. Iliacus muscle
33. Iliolumbar a. & v.
34. Internal iliac a. & v.
35. Deep circumflex iliac a.
36. Superior vesicle a.
37. Urinary bladder
38. Cremasteric a.
39. Obturator a.
40. Spermatic cord
41. Esophagus
42. Spleen
43. Aortic hiatus
44. Celiac trunk
45. Superior mesenteric a.
46. Left renal a. & v.
47. Ureter
48. Quadratus lumborum muscle
49. 4th lumbar a. & v.
50. Middle sacral a. & v.
51. Superior gluteal a. & v.
52. External iliac a. & v.
53. Inguinal ligament
54. Inferior epigastric a.
55. Superficial circumflex iliac a. & v.
56. External pudendal aa. & vv.
57. Internal pudendal a. & v.
58. Deep dorsal v. and dorsal a. of penis
59. Pampiniform venous plexus
60. Testicle

Branches of Abdominal Aorta and Portal Vein

Diaphragm
Right lobe of liver
Gallbladder
Pancreas
Duodenum
Ascending colon
Ileum
Cecum
Appendix
Falciform ligament
Left lobe of liver
Spleen
Stomach
Jejunum
Transverse colon
Descending colon
Sigmoid colon
Rectum
External anal sphincter muscle

Key: Vessels of Abdomen

1. Intercostal a. & v.
2. Azygos v.
3. Thoracic duct
4. Thoracic aorta
5. Hemiazygos v.
6. Esophageal venous plexus
7. Hepatic vv.
8. Inferior vena cava
9. Common hepatic duct
10. Proper hepatic a.
11. Cystic duct
12. Common bile duct
13. Gastroduodenal a.
14. Anterior superior pancreaticoduodenal a.
15. Pancreatic duct
16. Anterior inferior pancreaticoduodenal a.
17. Right colic a. & v.
18. Ileocolic a. & v.
19. Left gastric a. & v.
20. Short gastric aa. & vv.
21. Inferior phrenic a.
22. Celiac trunk
23. Common hepatic a.
24. Splenic a.
25. Cisterna chyli
26. Right gastric a.
27. Portal v.
28. Left gastroepiploic a. & vv.
29. Superior mesenteric a. & v.
30. Right gastroepiploic a. & v.
31. Middle colic a. & v.
32. Jejunal & ileal aa. & vv.
33. Inferior mesenteric a. & v.
34. Left colic a. & v.
35. Common iliac aa. & vv.
36. Sigmoid aa. & vv.
37. Middle sacral a. & v.
38. Superior rectal a. & v.
39. Right internal iliac a. & v.
40. Middle rectal a. & v.
41. Inferior rectal a. & v.

Key: Abbreviations

Artery – a.	Cervical vertebra – C
Arteries – aa.	Nerve – n.
Branch – br.	Vein – v.
Branches – brs.	Veins – vv.

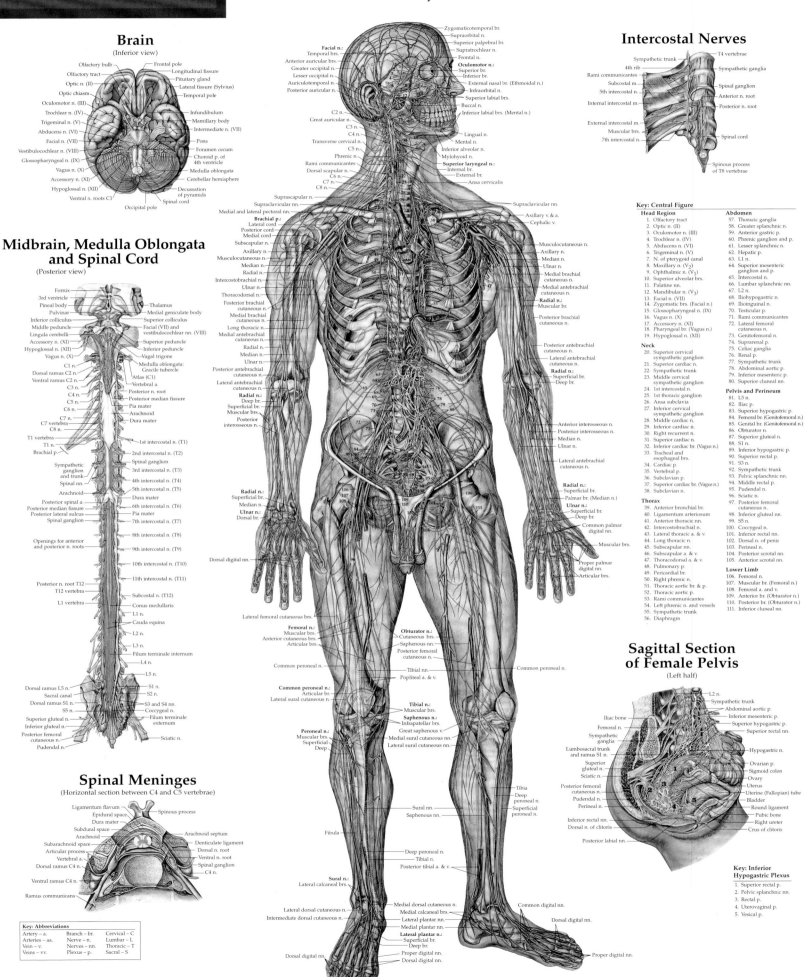

Brain
(Inferior view)

Olfactory bulb
Olfactory tract
Optic n. (II)
Optic chiasm
Oculomotor n. (III)
Trochlear n. (IV)
Trigeminal n. (V)
Abducens n. (VI)
Facial n. (VII)
Vestibulocochlear n. (VIII)
Glossopharyngeal n. (IX)
Vagus n. (X)
Accessory n. (XI)
Hypoglossal n. (XII)
Ventral n. roots C1

Frontal pole
Longitudinal fissure
Pituitary gland
Lateral fissure (Sylvius)
Temporal pole
Infundibulum
Mamillary body
Intermediate n. (VII)
Pons
Foramen cecum
Choroid p. of 4th ventricle
Medulla oblongata
Cerebellar hemisphere
Decussation of pyramids
Spinal cord
Occipital pole

Intercostal Nerves

Sympathetic trunk
4th rib
Rami communicantes
Subcostal n.
5th intercostal n.
Internal intercostal m.
External intercostal m.
7th intercostal n.
T4 vertebrae
Sympathetic ganglia
Spinal ganglion
Anterior n. root
Posterior n. root
Spinal cord
Muscular brs.
Spinous process of T8 vertebrae

Midbrain, Medulla Oblongata and Spinal Cord
(Posterior view)

Fornix
3rd ventricle
Pineal body
Pulvinar
Inferior colliculus
Middle peduncle
Lingula cerebelli
Accessory n. (XI)
Hypoglossal n. (XII)
Vagus n. (X)
C1 n.
Dorsal ramus C2 n.
Ventral ramus C2 n.
C3 n.
C4 n.
C5 n.
C6 n.
C7 vertebra
C8 n.
T1 vertebra
T1 n.
Brachial p.

Thalamus
Medial geniculate body
Superior colliculus
Facial (VII) and vestibulocochlear nn. (VIII)
Superior peduncle
Inferior peduncle
Vagal trigone
Medulla oblongata: Gracile tubercle
Atlas (C1)
Vertebral a.
Posterior n. root
Posterior median fissure
Pia mater
Arachnoid
Dura mater
1st intercostal n. (T1)
2nd intercostal n. (T2)
Spinal ganglion
3rd intercostal n. (T3)
Spinal n.

Sympathetic ganglion and trunk
Spinal n.
Arachnoid
Posterior spinal a.
Posterior median fissure
Posterior lateral sulcus
Spinal ganglion

Openings for anterior and posterior n. roots

Posterior n. root T12
T12 vertebra
L1 vertebra

4th intercostal n. (T4)
5th intercostal n. (T5)
Dura mater
6th intercostal n. (T6)
Pia mater
7th intercostal n. (T7)
8th intercostal n. (T8)
9th intercostal n. (T9)
10th intercostal n. (T10)
11th intercostal n. (T11)
Subcostal n. (T12)
Conus medullaris
Cauda equina
L2 n.
L3 n.
Filum terminale internum
L4 n.
L5 n.
S1 n.
S2 n.
S3 and S4 nn.
S5 n.
Coccygeal n.
Filum terminale externum

Dorsal ramus L5 n.
Sacral canal
Dorsal ramus S1 n.
S5 n.
Superior gluteal n.
Inferior gluteal n.
Posterior femoral cutaneous n.
Pudendal n.
Sciatic n.

Spinal Meninges
(Horizontal section between C4 and C5 vertebrae)

Ligamentum flavum
Epidural space
Dura mater
Subdural space
Arachnoid
Subarachnoid space
Articular process
Vertebral a.
Dorsal ramus C4 n.
Ventral ramus C4 n.
Ramus communicans

Spinous process
Arachnoid septum
Denticulate ligament
Dorsal n. root
Ventral n. root
Spinal ganglion
C4 n.

Key: Central Figure

Head Region
1. Olfactory tract
2. Optic n. (II)
3. Oculomotor n. (III)
4. Trochlear n. (IV)
5. Abducens n. (VI)
6. Trigeminal n. (V)
7. N. of pterygoid canal
8. Maxillary n. (V₂)
9. Ophthalmic n. (V₁)
10. Superior alveolar brs.
11. Palatine nn.
12. Mandibular n. (V₃)
13. Facial n. (VII)
14. Zygomatic brs. (Facial n.)
15. Glossopharyngeal n. (IX)
16. Vagus n. (X)
17. Accessory n. (XI)
18. Pharyngeal br. (Vagus n.)
19. Hypoglossal n. (XII)

Neck
20. Superior cervical sympathetic ganglion
21. Superior cardiac n.
22. Sympathetic trunk
23. Middle cervical sympathetic ganglion
24. 1st intercostal n.
25. 1st thoracic ganglion
26. Ansa subclavia
27. Inferior cervical sympathetic ganglion
28. Middle cardiac n.
29. Inferior cardiac n.
30. Right recurrent n.
31. Superior cardiac n.
32. Inferior cardiac br. (Vagus n.)
33. Tracheal and esophageal brs.
34. Cardiac p.
35. Vertebral p.
36. Subclavian a.
37. Superior cardiac br. (Vagus n.)
38. Subclavian v.

Thorax
39. Anterior bronchial br.
40. Ligamentum arteriosum
41. Anterior thoracic nn.
42. Intercostobrachial n.
43. Lateral thoracic a. & v.
44. Long thoracic n.
45. Subscapular nn.
46. Subscapular a. & v.
47. Thoracodorsal a. & v.
48. Pulmonary p.
49. Pericardial br.
50. Right phrenic n.
51. Thoracic aortic br. & p.
52. Thoracic aortic p.
53. Rami communicantes
54. Left phrenic n. and vessels
55. Sympathetic trunk
56. Diaphragm

Abdomen
57. Thoracic ganglia
58. Greater splanchnic n.
59. Anterior gastric p.
60. Phrenic ganglion and p.
61. Lesser splanchnic n.
62. Hepatic p.
63. L1 n.
64. Superior mesenteric ganglion and p.
65. Intercostal n.
66. Lumbar splanchnic nn.
67. L2 n.
68. Iliohypogastric n.
69. Ilioinguinal n.
70. Testicular p.
71. Rami communicantes
72. Lateral femoral cutaneous n.
73. Genitofemoral n.
74. Suprarenal p.
75. Celiac ganglia
76. Renal p.
77. Sympathetic trunk
78. Abdominal aortic p.
79. Inferior mesenteric p.
80. Superior cluneal n.

Pelvis and Perineum
81. L5 n.
82. Iliac p.
83. Superior hypogastric p.
84. Femoral br. (Genitofemoral n.)
85. Genital br. (Genitofemoral n.)
86. Obturator n.
87. Superior gluteal n.
88. S1 n.
89. Inferior hypogastric p.
90. Superior rectal p.
91. S3 n.
92. Sympathetic trunk
93. Pelvic splanchnic nn.
94. Middle rectal p.
95. Pudendal n.
96. Sciatic n.
97. Posterior femoral cutaneous n.
98. Inferior gluteal nn.
99. S5 n.
100. Coccygeal n.
101. Inferior rectal nn.
102. Dorsal n. of penis
103. Perineal n.
104. Posterior scrotal nn.
105. Anterior scrotal nn.

Lower Limb
106. Femoral n.
107. Muscular br. (Femoral n.)
108. Femoral a. and v.
109. Anterior br. (Obturator n.)
110. Posterior br. (Obturator n.)
111. Inferior cluneal nn.

Sagittal Section of Female Pelvis
(Left half)

L2 n.
Sympathetic trunk
Abdominal aortic p.
Inferior mesenteric p.
Superior hypogastric p.
Superior rectal nn.
Iliac bone
Femoral n.
Sympathetic ganglia
Lumbosacral trunk and ramus S1 n.
Superior gluteal n.
Sciatic n.
Posterior femoral cutaneous n.
Pudendal n.
Perineal n.
Inferior rectal nn.
Dorsal n. of clitoris
Posterior labial nn.

Hypogastric p.
Ovarian p.
Sigmoid colon
Ovary
Uterus
Uterine (Fallopian) tube
Bladder
Round ligament
Right ureter
Pubic bone
Crus of clitoris

Key: Inferior Hypogastric Plexus
1. Superior rectal p.
2. Pelvic splanchnic p.
3. Rectal p.
4. Uterovaginal p.
5. Vesical p.

Key: Abbreviations
Artery – a.	Branch – br.	Cervical – C
Arteries – aa.	Nerve – n.	Lumbar – L
Vein – v.	Nerves – nn.	Thoracic – T
Veins – vv.	Plexus – p.	Sacral – S

(Central figure labels include: Facial n.: Temporal brs., Zygomaticotemporal br., Supraorbital n., Superior palpebral br., Supratrochlear n., Frontal n., Anterior auricular brs., Oculomotor n.: Superior br., Inferior br., Greater occipital n., Lesser occipital n., Auriculotemporal n., Posterior auricular n., External nasal br. (Ethmoidal n.), Infraorbital n., Superior labial brs., Buccal n., Inferior labial brs. (Mental n.), C2 n., Great auricular n., C3 n., Lingual n., C4 n., Mental n., Transverse cervical n., Inferior alveolar n., Phrenic n., Mylohyoid n., Rami communicantes, Superior laryngeal n.: Internal br., External br., Dorsal scapular n., Ansa cervicalis, C6 n., C7 n., C8 n., Suprascapular n., Supraclavicular nn., Medial and lateral pectoral nn., Brachial p.: Lateral cord, Posterior cord, Medial cord, Subscapular n., Axillary n., Musculocutaneous n., Median n., Radial n., Intercostobrachial n., Ulnar n., Thoracodorsal n., Posterior brachial cutaneous n., Medial brachial cutaneous n., Long thoracic n., Medial antebrachial cutaneous n., Radial n., Median n., Ulnar n., Posterior antebrachial cutaneous n., Lateral antebrachial cutaneous n., Radial n.: Deep br., Superficial br., Muscular brs., Posterior interosseous n., Radial n.: Superficial br., Median n., Ulnar n.: Dorsal br., Dorsal digital nn., Musculocutaneous n., Median n., Ulnar n., Medial brachial cutaneous n., Medial antebrachial cutaneous n., Radial n.: Muscular br., Posterior brachial cutaneous n., Posterior antebrachial cutaneous n., Lateral antebrachial cutaneous n., Radial n.: Superficial br., Deep br., Anterior interosseous n., Posterior interosseous n., Median n., Ulnar n., Lateral antebrachial cutaneous n., Radial n.: Superficial br., Palmar br. (Median n.), Ulnar n.: Superficial br., Deep br., Common palmar digital nn., Muscular brs., Proper palmar digital nn., Articular brs., Axillary v. & a., Cephalic v., Musculocutaneous n., Median n., Ulnar n., Medial brachial cutaneous n., Medial antebrachial cutaneous n., Lateral femoral cutaneous brs., Femoral n.: Muscular brs., Anterior cutaneous brs., Articular brs., Common peroneal n., Obturator n.: Cutaneous brs., Saphenous nn., Posterior femoral cutaneous n., Tibial nn., Popliteal a. & v., Common peroneal n., Common peroneal n.: Articular br., Lateral sural cutaneous n., Tibial n.: Muscular brs., Saphenous n.: Infrapatellar brs., Great saphenous v., Medial sural cutaneous nn., Lateral sural cutaneous nn., Peroneal n.: Muscular brs., Superficial, Deep, Tibia, Deep peroneal n., Tibial n., Posterior tibial a. & v., Sural nn., Saphenous nn., Fibula, Deep peroneal n., Tibial n., Posterior tibial a. & v., Sural n.: Lateral calcaneal brs., Lateral dorsal cutaneous n., Intermediate dorsal cutaneous n., Medial dorsal cutaneous n., Medial calcaneal brs., Lateral plantar nn., Medial plantar nn., Lateral plantar n.: Superficial br., Deep br., Proper digital nn., Dorsal digital nn., Common digital nn., Dorsal digital nn., Proper digital nn.)

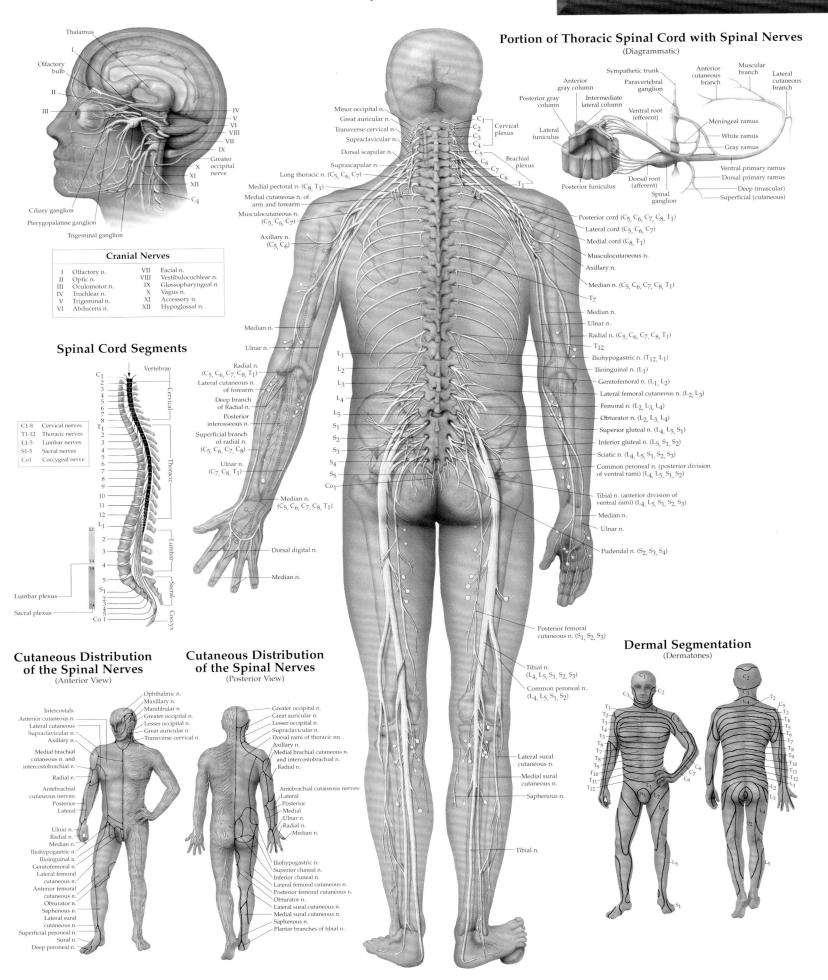

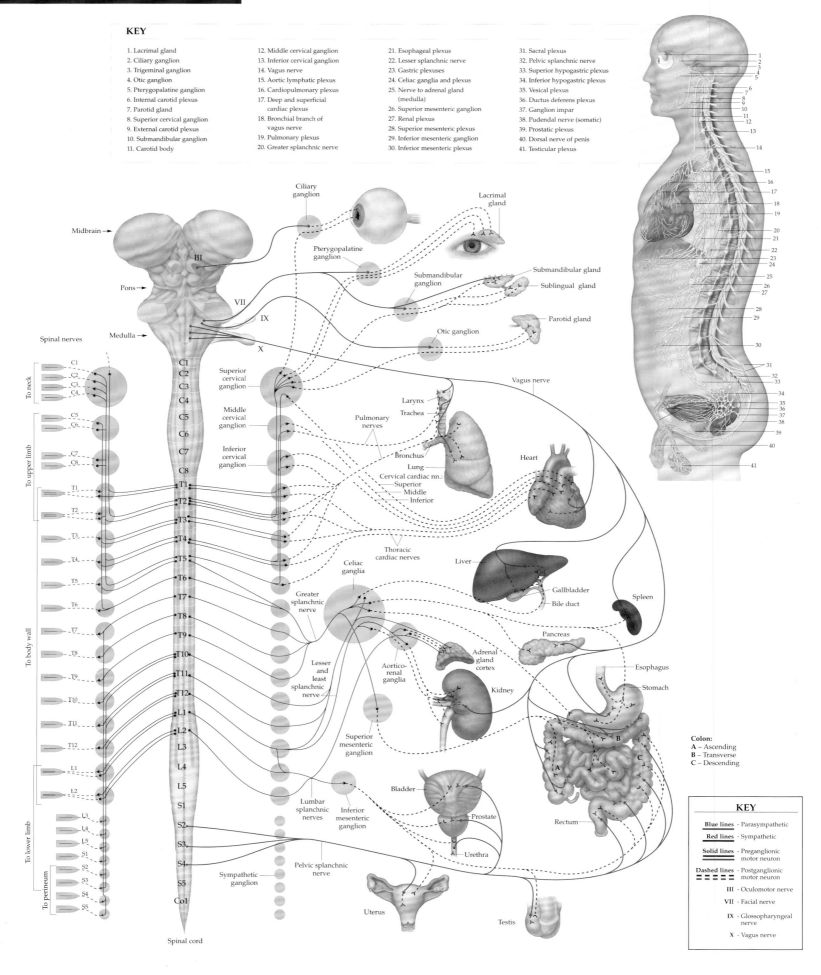

KEY

1. Lacrimal gland
2. Ciliary ganglion
3. Trigeminal ganglion
4. Otic ganglion
5. Pterygopalatine ganglion
6. Internal carotid plexus
7. Parotid gland
8. Superior cervical ganglion
9. External carotid plexus
10. Submandibular ganglion
11. Carotid body
12. Middle cervical ganglion
13. Inferior cervical ganglion
14. Vagus nerve
15. Aortic lymphatic plexus
16. Cardiopulmonary plexus
17. Deep and superficial cardiac plexus
18. Bronchial branch of vagus nerve
19. Pulmonary plexus
20. Greater splanchnic nerve
21. Esophageal plexus
22. Lesser splanchnic nerve
23. Gastric plexuses
24. Celiac ganglia and plexus
25. Nerve to adrenal gland (medulla)
26. Superior mesenteric ganglion
27. Renal plexus
28. Superior mesenteric plexus
29. Inferior mesenteric ganglion
30. Inferior mesenteric plexus
31. Sacral plexus
32. Pelvic splanchnic nerve
33. Superior hypogastric plexus
34. Inferior hypogastric plexus
35. Vesical plexus
36. Ductus deferens plexus
37. Ganglion impar
38. Pudendal nerve (somatic)
39. Prostatic plexus
40. Dorsal nerve of penis
41. Testicular plexus

Colon:
A – Ascending
B – Transverse
C – Descending

KEY

Blue lines - Parasympathetic
Red lines - Sympathetic
Solid lines - Preganglionic motor neuron
Dashed lines - Postganglionic motor neuron
III - Oculomotor nerve
VII - Facial nerve
IX - Glossopharyngeal nerve
X - Vagus nerve

Index

Anatomical Visual Guide to Sports Injuries